Placental, Neonatal, and Pediatric Pathology

Placental, Neonatal, and Pediatric Pathology

Based on the Proceedings of the Sixty-First Annual Anatomic Pathology Slide Seminar of the American Society of Clinical Pathologists

September 21 and 22, 1995
New Orleans, Louisiana

PRELECTORS

DON B. SINGER, MD
Pathologist-in-Chief
Women and Infants Hospital
Professor of Pathology
Brown University
School of Medicine
Providence, Rhode Island

LOUIS P. DEHNER, MD
Director, Division of Anatomic Pathology
Professor of Pathology
Washington University Medical Center
St Louis, Missouri

MODERATOR

YAO SHI FU, MD
Professor of Pathology
Chief of Surgical Pathology
University of California at Los Angeles Medical Center
Los Angeles, California

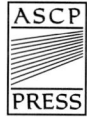

American Society of Clinical Pathologists
Chicago

Library of Congress Cataloging-in-Publication Data

Anatomic Pathology Slide Seminar (61st: 1995: New Orleans, La.)
  Placental, neonatal, and pediatric pathology: based on the proceedings of the Sixty-First Annual Anatomic Pathology Slide Seminar of the American Society of Clinical Pathologists, September 21 and 22, 1995, New Orleans, Louisiana/ prelectors, Don B. Singer, Louis P. Dehner; moderator, Yao Shi Fu.
       p.   cm.
  Includes bibliographical references.
  ISBN 0-89189-404-7 (alk. paper)
  1. Pediatric pathology—Case studies—Slides—Congresses. 2. Placenta—Histopathology—Case studies—Slides—Congresses. 3. Anatomy, Pathological—Case studies—Slides—Congresses.
  I. Singer, Don B. II. Dehner, Louis P., 1940- . III. Fu, Yao S. IV. American Society of Clinical Pathologists. V. Title.
  [DNLM: 1. Placenta Diseases—pathology—congresses. 2. Fetal Diseases—pathology—congresses. 4. Pediatrics—congresses. WQ 212 A535 1996]
FJ49.A53   1995
618.92'007—dc20
DNLM/DLC
for Library of Congress   96-620
                                                                                                           CIP

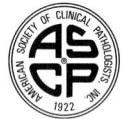

Copyright © 1996 by the American Society of Clinical Pathologists. All rights reserved. No part of this publication may be reproduced, stored in a retrieval system, or transmitted in any form or by any means, electronic, mechanical, photocopying, recording or otherwise, without the prior written permission of the publisher.

Printed in the United States of America.

00 99 98 97 96   5 4 3 2 1

Contents

Foreword   vii

Case 1.   Chronic villitis of unknown etiology   1

Case 2.   Acute fetal listeriosis with diffuse acute villitis and miliary micro-abscesses   8

Case 3.   Inflammatory myofibroblastic tumor of the jejunum   13

Case 4.   Fibrous hamartoma of infancy   21

Case 5.   Fetal infection with excessive granulopoiesis in the liver; a leukemoid reaction or transient abnormal myelopoiesis (TAM)   26

Case 6.   Fetal parvovirus B19 infection   31

Case 7.   Alpers-like syndrome with micronodular cirrhosis and leuko-encephalopathy   38

Case 8.   Undifferentiated (embryonal) sarcoma of the liver   45

Case 9.   Neonatal coxsackievirus B1 infection   53

Case 10.   Foregut cyst   60

Case 11.   Angiomyolipoma, renal cell carcinoma, and multiple cysts of the kidney   65

Case 12.   Wilms' tumor of the kidney with postchemotherapy changes and bilateral nephroblastomatosis   75

Case 13.   Ivemark's renal-hepatic-pancreatic dysplasia   83

Case 14.   Juvenile polyposis coli   92

Case 15.   Sclerosing stromal tumor of the ovary   98

Case 16.   Adult type granulosa cell tumor, macrofollicular variant   103

Case 17.   Friedreich's ataxia   108

Case 18.   Thyroid hyperplasia in boy with undiagnosed thyrotoxicosis and thyroid storm   113

Case 19.   Malignant rhabdoid (pseudorhabdoid) tumor   119

Case 20.   Soft tissue Ewing's sarcoma of the vulva   126

Foreword

The 61st Annual Anatomic Pathology Slide Seminar of the American Society of Clinical Pathologists (ASCP) was held on September 21 and 22, 1995, in New Orleans, Louisiana. The prelectors of the seminar were Don B. Singer, MD, and Louis P. Dehner, MD, with myself as moderator. The Society was most fortunate to have two distinguished teachers and well-known authorities to conduct this seminar on placental, neonatal, and pediatric pathology. This kind of combined seminar has never been held before and reflects the remarkable changes in the fields in the last 15 years, such as increased molecular information, development of novel diagnostic techniques, and recent discoveries of disease entities.

Using carefully selected cases, Drs Singer and Dehner led the audience to explore placental pathology, an area whose importance is often ignored by most residency training programs and in which most pathologists are less than optimally informed. Following the placenta, key models of neoplastic and non-neoplastic diseases of newborns and pediatric patients were discussed from the viewpoints of diagnostic features, differential diagnosis, and use of immunohistochemical and genetic markers to achieve optimal diagnosis. In spite of the rarity of some of the cases, the audience was rewarded with practical, first-hand experience that was enhanced by beautiful slides and humorous remarks. Both prelectors demonstrated their vast knowledge of the subject and convinced the participants of the clinical relevance of the correct diagnosis. All those present at the seminar, although at times overwhelmed by the new scientific data, considered the time well spent and the slide seminar a great success.

The first speaker, Dr Singer, graduated from Baylor College of Medicine, Houston, Texas, and received his residency training at Boston Children's Hospital, New England Deaconess Hospital, and Stanford University Hospital, Palo Alto, California. This was followed by a faculty position in the Department of Pathology at his alma mater. Since 1975, Dr Singer has been Professor of Pathology at Brown University School of Medicine, where he is also Director of the Developmental Pathology Program. Dr Singer is currently Pathologist-in-Chief at Women and Infants' Hospital, Providence, Rhode Island, and Staff Pathologist at Rhode Island Hospital. He serves on major hospital and university committees and holds offices in key professional societies. His numerous original contributions and textbooks, including *Forensic Aspects in Pediatric Pathology* (Karger, Basel; 1995), *Human Reproduction: Growth and Development* (Little, Brown Co, Boston; 1995), and *Textbook of Fetal and Perinatal Pathology* (Blackwell Scientific Publications, Boston; 1991) are widely referenced and greatly admired.

The second speaker, Dr Dehner, grew up in St Louis and received his bachelor's degree, medical degree, and pathology training all at Washington University and Barnes Hospital, where he is currently Professor of Pathology and Pediatrics, Director of Anatomic Pathology and Surgical Pathologist-in-Chief, and Pathologist-in-Chief at St Louis Children's Hospital. Dr Dehner receives many honors as visiting professor and invited lecturer worldwide, serves on multiple hospital and university committees, contributes to the editorial boards of and holds offices in the professional societies. His comprehensive textbooks *Pediatric Surgical Pathology* (Williams & Wilkins, Baltimore; 1987) and *Pediatric Pathology* (Lippincott, Philadelphia; 1992) and numerous original observations and book chapters have made major impacts on our daily practice of pediatric and surgical pathology.

As the moderator of this prestigious ASCP Anatomic Pathology Slide Seminar, I would like to acknowledge the dedication and support of my capable ASCP officers and staff members, especially Robert C. Rock, MD, Senior Vice President; Kathy Mauck, MT(ASCP); Sondra Moran, MT(ASCP); Lynn Zieger, MT(ASCP); and the histotechnologists at the ASCP headquarters in Chicago. Their assistance, combined with the efforts of Drs Singer and Dehner, made this slide seminar one of the most memorable events in the series.

Yao S. Fu, MD

Case One

Contributed by Don B. Singer, MD
Providence, Rhode Island

History

A 38-year-old woman in her ninth pregnancy presented 2 years previously with an intrauterine device that was embedded in the endometrium and removed with great difficulty. Following this, her seventh and eighth pregnancies ended in early spontaneous abortions. This placenta is from a 38-week gestation. Her 4-year-old son had chickenpox; her varicella IgG titer was 1:75.

Dr Singer: The placenta has small groups and larger collections of inflammatory cells, predominantly in the intervillous space but also invading some of the villi (Figure 1-1). Most of the cells are macrophages, mixed with neutrophils and occasional lymphocytes and eosinophils. Plasma cells are notably absent. Where the villous surface is breached, the overlying syncytial trophoblast is eroded (Figure 1-2). Fibrin deposits are rare and extend minimally into the intervillous space. Many villi are fibrotic and some show early reparative change with plump fibroblasts (Figure 1-3). The membranes and fetal surfaces of the placenta are meconium stained and meconium macrophages extend deep into the chorion. This is an example of intervillositis and chronic villitis of undetermined etiology (VUE) with meconium staining.

Some general comments regarding the importance of placental examination should be considered. As stated by Gillan,[1] the placenta may be viewed as a diary of the pregnancy. It audits antenatal clinical judgment by clinicopathologic correlation. It makes a contribution in the context of unsolved clinical problems. Because it occupies the interface of fetus and mother, the merged images cause confusion. The last comment applies especially well to VUE, an interesting and puzzling condition.

The importance of focal and multifocal chronic villitis was first emphasized by Benirschke and Altshuler in 1971.[2] Altshuler coined the term *villitis of unknown etiology* in 1973.[3] One of the largest series of placentas evaluated for this lesion was reported by Russell, who examined 7,505 placentas and found VUE in 570 (7.6%).[4] The spectrum of severity and distribution of lesions was from very mild and focal villitis to intense and widely distributed chronic villitis. Altshuler and Russell delineated several types of villitis, designating them proliferative, necrotizing, exudative, granulomatous, and chronic forms.[5-7] In VUE, the inflammatory cells are mostly macrophages, T-helper lymphocytes, and some polymorphonuclear white blood cells.[8] Although Benirschke and Kaufmann[9] speculated that the macrophages are of fetal origin, others have shown that virtually all are derived from the mother.[10] Redline and Patterson,

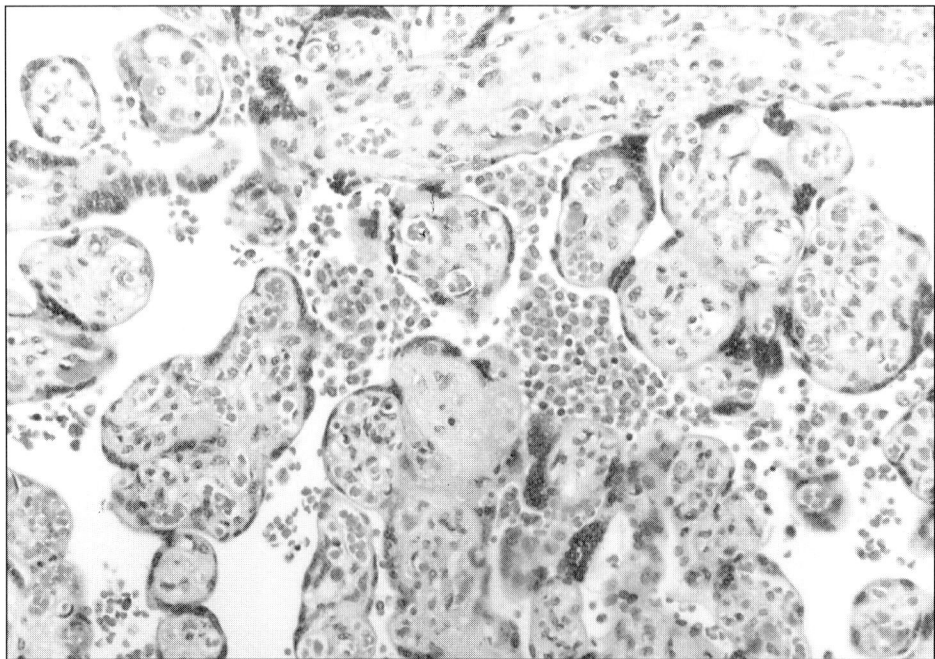

Figure 1–1. Villitis and intervillositis. The cells are mostly macrophages with lymphocytes and a few neutrophils and eosinophils.

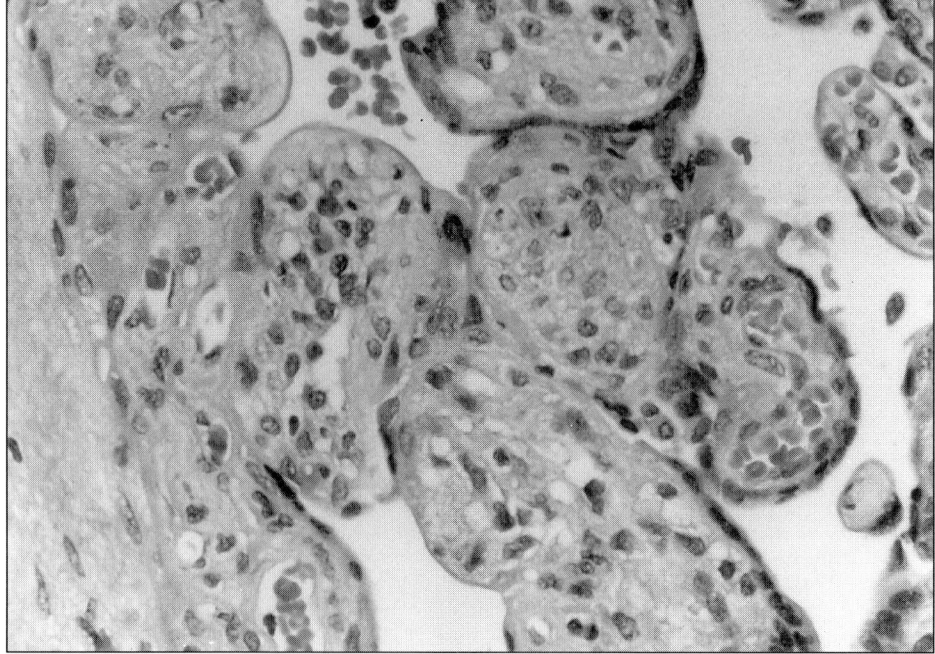

Figure 1–2. Villitis of unknown etiology with mononuclear inflammation of villous stroma. The syncytial trophoblast is eroded or destroyed with minimal fibrin deposits.

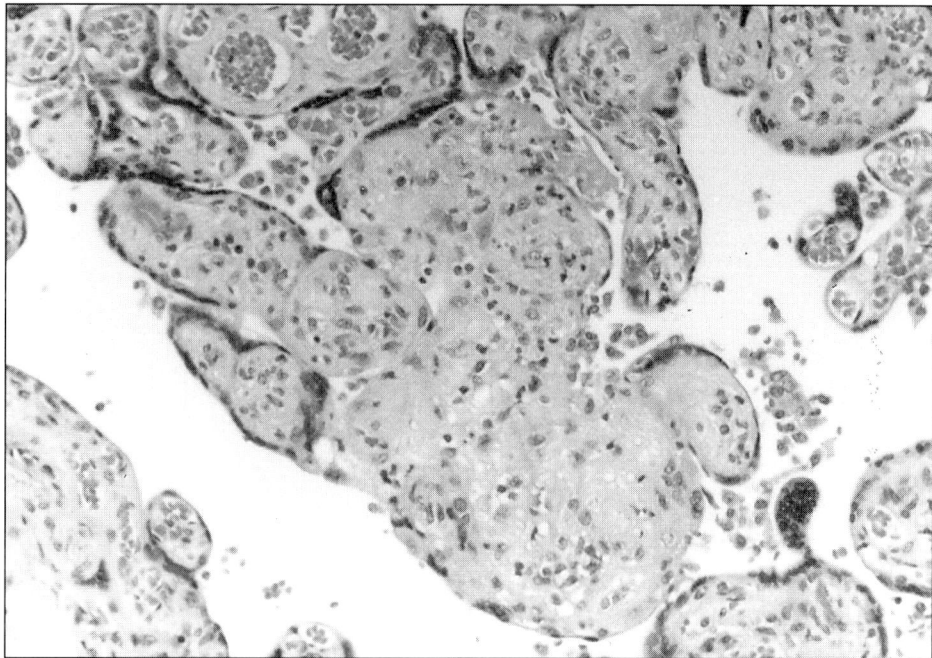

Figure 1–3. Some of the villi are fibrotic, suggesting a healing phase.

using a Y-chromosome probe in placentas from male babies, demonstrated that the inflammatory cells in VUE were negative for Y antigen.[11] B-Lymphocytes and plasma cells are usually absent. Mononuclear cells have HLA-DR antigen in 75% of cases, but HLA-DP and HLA-DQ antigens are also present.[12]

Khong et al conducted a survey to determine the consistency with which experienced pathologists diagnosed VUE.[13] Fifty slides of placental tissue were submitted to three pathologists; then the same 50 slides plus 20 more were sent to the same three pathologists. Intraobserver agreement for the presence of VUE was 85% and interobserver agreement was 81%. Most of the disagreements occurred in cases of focal VUE. While the authors concluded that agreement was relatively poor, these results surpassed interobserver agreement in similar surveys regarding borderline epithelial lesions of the breast[14,15] and prostatic lesions.[16]

Other placental lesions associated with VUE include chronic chorioamnionitis, infarcts, avascular villi, vasculitis, necrotizing deciduitis, necrotizing funisitis, chorangiosis, and extensive fibrin deposits especially surrounding and choking villi close to the decidua basalis, the so-called maternal floor infarct.[9,17–20]

Infections that are not associated with VUE include acute chorioamnionitis due to bacterial infections,[21,22] HIV infections,[23] and cryptococcal infection.[24] Rubella infection produces an endovascular lesion in the villi but no inflammatory infiltrate.[25] Hemorrhagic endovasculitis has no associated villitis.[26]

Are the lesions in this case different from VUE? We found a predominantly intervillous collection of mononuclear cells, ie, an intervillositis. Intervillositis occurs in about 1 in 500 placentas, while VUE is much more common, occurring in about 1 in 10 placentas.[27] Intervillositis is associated with more intervillous fibrinoid material and trophoblast necrosis than is VUE. Intrauterine growth retardation is more consistently a feature of intervillositis than it is of VUE. In the series reported by Jacques and Qureshi, five of six cases of intervillositis ended with perinatal death.[27] In our case, while the intervillous inflammatory cells are prominent, sufficient invasion of villi is present to favor the diagnosis of villitis over intervillositis.

Villitis of unknown etiology is associated with many clinical conditions. Most commonly mentioned is intrauterine growth retardation, often repeating in subsequent pregnancies.[6,9,17,28-30] According to Nordenvall and Sandstedt, the extent of villous inflammation correlates with the degree of growth failure.[31] Despite this, about one fourth of the cases are found with babies of normal size,[32] and in our case the baby has grown normally and is thriving at 2 years of age. Other associated clinical findings with VUE include twinning,[33] coagulation disorders,[34] and a number of nonhypertensive conditions.[17] Since IgM concentrations are not elevated in the sera of mothers or babies, maternal and fetal infections, other than those mentioned below, are apparently unassociated with the lesions seen in VUE.[32]

Once the diagnosis of chronic villitis is established, an effort must be made to identify the few known infectious causes. These comprise the major differential diagnoses and include cytomegalovirus infection,[35,36] syphilis,[37-39] toxoplasmosis,[40,41] and varicella.[42,43] The diagnosis of these infectious agents can be enhanced with special techniques such as immunohistochemistry or in situ hybridization using molecular probes.[36] We recently examined a placenta from a mother who was exposed to varicella at about 13 weeks' gestation. The fetal tissues had foci with intranuclear inclusions that stained positively with anti-varicella/zoster immunohistochemical stains. The placenta had a diffuse intense necrotizing chronic villitis. Greco et al[8] found that both cytomegalovirus (CMV) villitis and VUE have intense reactivity to macrophage markers. Schwartz et al,[44] who studied placentas with known CMV, found marked hyperplasia of Hofbauer cells and lymphocytic villitis. In our case, a sibling had varicella at the time of this baby's delivery, but the mother was immune, and immunohistochemical stains of the placenta for varicella, CMV, and herpes were negative.

In VUE, immunologic reactions comprise a possible group of pathogenetic mechanisms.[12,30,45] Term placentas have no class II MHC antigens in the normal syncytiotrophoblast, but in areas with VUE, fetal stem vessels demonstrate class II MHC antigen.[12] Studies such as these have not been independently confirmed, although others have speculated that VUE is an immunologically mediated lesion.[46] In most cases, the etiology is unknown and the designation *villitis of undetermined etiology* (VUE) is appropriate.

DIAGNOSIS: Chronic villitis of unknown etiology

References

1. Gillan JE. Perinatal placental pathology. *Curr Opinion Obstet Gynecol* 1992;4: 286-294.
2. Benirschke K, Altshuler G. The future of perinatal physiopathology. In: Abramson H, ed. *Symposium on the Functional Physiopathology of the Fetus and Neonate.* St Louis: CV Mosby; 1971:158-168.
3. Altshuler G. Placental villitis of unknown etiology: Harbinger of serious disease? A four months' experience of nine cases. *J Reprod Med* 1973;11:215-222.
4. Russell P. Inflammatory lesions of the human placenta. III. The histopathology of villitis of unknown aetiology. *Placenta* 1980;1:227-244.
5. Altshuler G, Russell P. The human placental villitides: A review of chronic intrauterine infection. *Curr Top Pathol* 1975;60:64-112.
6. Altshuler G. Proceedings: Continuing experience of placental villitis of unknown aetiology: harbinger of serious disease? *Arch Dis Childhood* 1975;50:662.
7. Altshuler G. Placentitis, with a new light on an old TORCH. *Obstet Gynecol Annu* 1977;6:197-211.
8. Greco MA, Wieczorek R, Sachdev R, Kaplan C, Nuovo GJ, Demopoulos RI. Phenotype of villous stromal cells in placentas with cytomegalovirus, syphilis, and nonspecific villitis. *Am J Pathol* 1992;141:835-842.
9. Benirschke K, Kaufmann P. *Pathology of the Human Placenta.* 2nd ed. New York: Springer-Verlag: 1990;606-613.
10. Altemani AM. Immunohistochemical study of the inflammatory infiltrate in villitis of unknown etiology: A qualitative and quantitative analysis. *Pathol Res Pract* 1992;188:303-309.
11. Redline RW, Patterson P. Villitis of unknown etiology is associated with major infiltration of fetal tissue by maternal inflammatory cells. *Am J Pathol* 1993;143:473-479.
12. Labarrere CA, McIntyre JA, Faulk WP. Immunohistologic evidence that villitis in human normal term placentas is an immunologic lesion. *Am J Obstet Gynecol* 1990;162:515-522.
13. Khong TY, Staples A, Moore L, Byard RW. Observer reliability in assessing villitis of unknown aetiology. *J Clin Pathol* 1993;46:208-210.
14. Rosai J. Borderline epithelial lesions of the breast. *Am J Surg Pathol* 1991;15:209-221.
15. Schnitt SJ, Connolly JL, Tavassoli FA, et al. Interobserver reproducibility in the diagnosis of ductal proliferative breast lesions using standardized criteria. *Am J Surg Pathol* 1992;16:1133-1143.
16. Epstein JI, Grignon DJ, Humphrey PA, et al. Interobserver reproducibility in the diagnosis of prostatic intraepithelial neoplasia. *Am J Surg Pathol* 1995;19:873-886.
17. Redline RW, Patterson P. Patterns of placental injury: Correlations with gestational age, placental weight, and clinical diagnoses. *Arch Pathol Lab Med*

18. Gersell DJ. Chronic villitis, chronic chorioamnionitis, and maternal floor infarction. *Semin Diagn Pathol* 1993;10:251-266.
19. Jacques SM, Qureshi F. Necrotizing funisitis: A study of 45 cases. *Hum Pathol* 1992;23:1278-1283.
20. Gersell DJ, Phillips NJ. Chronic chorioamnionitis: A clinicopathologic study of 17 cases. *Int J Gynecol Pathol* 1991;10:217-229.
21. Ilagan NB, Elias EG, Liang KC, Kazzi G, Piligian J, Khatib G. Perinatal and neonatal significance of bacteria-related placental villous edema. *Acta Obstet Gynecol Scand* 1990;69:287-290.
22. Shen-Schwarz S, Ruchelli E, Brown D. Villous oedema of the placenta: A clinicopathological study. *Placenta* 1989;10:297-307.
23. Martin AW, Brady K, Smith SI, et al. Immunohistochemical localization of human immunodeficiency virus p24 antigen in placental tissue. *Human Pathol* 1992;23:411-414.
24. Molnar-Nadasdy G, Haesly I, Reed J, Altshuler G. Placental cryptococcosis in a mother with systemic lupus erythematosus. *Arch Pathol Lab Med* 1994;118:757-759.
25. Driscoll SG. Histopathology of gestational rubella. *Am J Dis Child* 1969;118: 49-53.
26. Shen-Schwarz S, Macpherson TA, Mueller-Heubach E. The clinical significance of hemorrhagic endovasculitis of the placenta. *Am J Obstet Gynecol* 1988;159:48-51.
27. Jacques SM, Qureshi F. Chronic intervillositis of the placenta. *Arch Pathol Lab Med* 1993;117:1032-1035.
28. Salafia CM, Vintzileos AM, Silberman L, Bantham KF, Vogel CA. Placental pathology of idiopathic intrauterine growth retardation at term. *Am J Perinatol* 1992;9:179-184.
29. Labarrere C, Althabe O, Telenta M. Chorionic villitis of unknown aetiology in placentae of idiopathic small for gestational age infants. *Placenta* 1982;3:309-318.
30. Labarrere C, Althabe O, Caletti E, Muscolo D. Deficiency of blocking factors in intrauterine growth retardation and its relationship with chronic villitis. *Am J Reprod Immunol Microbiol* 1986;10:14-19.
31. Nordenvall M, Sandstedt B. Placental villitis and intrauterine growth retardation in a Swedish population. *Acta Pathol Microbiol Immunol Scand* 1990;98:19-24.
32. Altemani AM, Fassoni A, Marba S. Cord IgM levels in placentas with villitis of unknown etiology. *J Perinat Med* 1989;17:465-468.
33. Jacques SM, Qureshi F. Chronic villitis of unknown etiology in twin gestations. *Pediatr Pathol* 1994;14:575-584.
34. Redline RW, Pappin A. Fetal thrombotic vasculopathy: The clinical significance of extensive avascular villi. *Hum Pathol* 1995;26:80-85.
35. Becroft DMO. Prenatal cytomegalovirus infection: Epidemiology, pathology, and pathogenesis. *Perspect Pediatr Pathol* 1981;6:203-241.
36. Sachdev R, Nuovo GJ, Kaplan C, Greco MA. In situ hybridization analysis for cytomegalovirus in chronic villitis. *Pediatr Pathol* 1990;10:909-917.
37. Oppenheimer EH, Dahms B. Congenital syphilis in the fetus and neonate. *Perspect Pediatr Pathol* 1981;6:115-138.

38. Qureshi F, Jacques SM, Reyes MP. Placental histopathology in syphilis. *Human Pathol* 1993;24:779-784.
39. Samson GR, Meyer MP, Blake DR, Cohen MC, Mouton SC. Syphilitic placentitis: An immunopathy. *Placenta* 1994;15:67-77.
40. Popek EJ. Granulomatous villitis due to *Toxoplasma gondii*. *Pediatr Pathol* 1992;12:281-288.
41. Dische MR, Gooch WM III. Congenital toxoplasmosis. *Perspect Pediatr Pathol* 1981;6:83-113.
42. Garcia AGP. Fetal infection in chickenpox and alastrum with histopathologic study of the placenta. *Pediatrics* 1963;32:895-901.
43. Robertson NJ, McKeever PA. Fetal and placental pathology in two cases of maternal varicella infection. *Pediatr Pathol* 1992;12:545-550.
44. Schwartz DA, Khan R, Stoll B. Characterization of the fetal inflammatory response to cytomegalovirus placentitis: An immunohistochemical study. *Arch Pathol Lab Med* 1992;116:21-27.
45. Faulk WP, Labarrere CA. HIV proteins in normal human placentae. *Am J Reprod Immunol* 1991;25:99-104.
46. Redline RW, Abramowsky CR. Clinical and pathological aspects of recurrent villitis. *Hum Pathol* 1985;16:727-731.

Case Two

Contributed by Don B. Singer, MD
Providence, Rhode Island

History

This male fetus was stillborn at 27 weeks' gestation. The mother was 34 years old. This, her fourth pregnancy, was uncomplicated until severe headache and generalized muscular aches developed 1 month prior to delivery. These symptoms subsided spontaneously after 1 week and the pregnancy continued for 3 more weeks. Fetal death was diagnosed when the mother noted decreased fetal movement.

Dr Singer: The diagnosis can be suspected from examination of the placenta, which has widespread microabscesses in the villi and acute diffuse chorioamnionitis (Figures 2–1 and 2–2). Such widespread involvement was at one time considered virtually pathognomonic for listeriosis.[1,2] While *Listeria monocytogenes* remains the first consideration for a causative agent, we now know that other bacteria and viruses can produce similar placental lesions. We have seen several examples of acute suppurative villitis due to staphylococci, *Haemophilus influenzae, Escherichia coli,* and group B streptococcus (Figure 2–3). A recent case of fetal varicella infection had similar lesions, but the infiltrate had more mononuclear cells than neutrophils. No doubt other organisms responsible for acute fetal/neonatal sepsis can also produce an acute villitis, but listerial infection should be at the top of the list of differential diagnoses when this lesion is found. Macroabscesses, as well as microabscesses, are found in the placenta in severe listeric infections (Figure 2–4). The macroabscesses may measure up to 3 cm and are usually multiple. They may be mistaken for ischemic infarcts, but larger ones have central cavitations.[3]

The first case of neonatal listeriosis was reported by Burn in 1935.[4] Since then, fetal and neonatal infections have been recognized sporadically and in small epidemics, most of which are related to ingestion of contaminated foodstuffs. Unpasteurized dairy products such as soft cheese have been the source of several outbreaks.[5] Incompletely pasteurized milk was blamed in one epidemic,[6] and a bottle of contaminated mineral oil was involved in another.[7] Raw vegetables and coleslaw have also been the source of outbreaks.[8] Of all cases of listeric infections in the United States, more than one third are in fetuses or infants less than 1 month of age. Neonates with listeriosis have higher circulating colony-stimulating factor-1 levels and subsequently higher monocyte counts than those of both noninfected newborns and newborns infected with nonlisteric organisms.[9]

Puerperal infections in the mother are rare but a flulike illness, such as in this case, often precedes delivery of an infected fetus or newborn infant. Clinically,

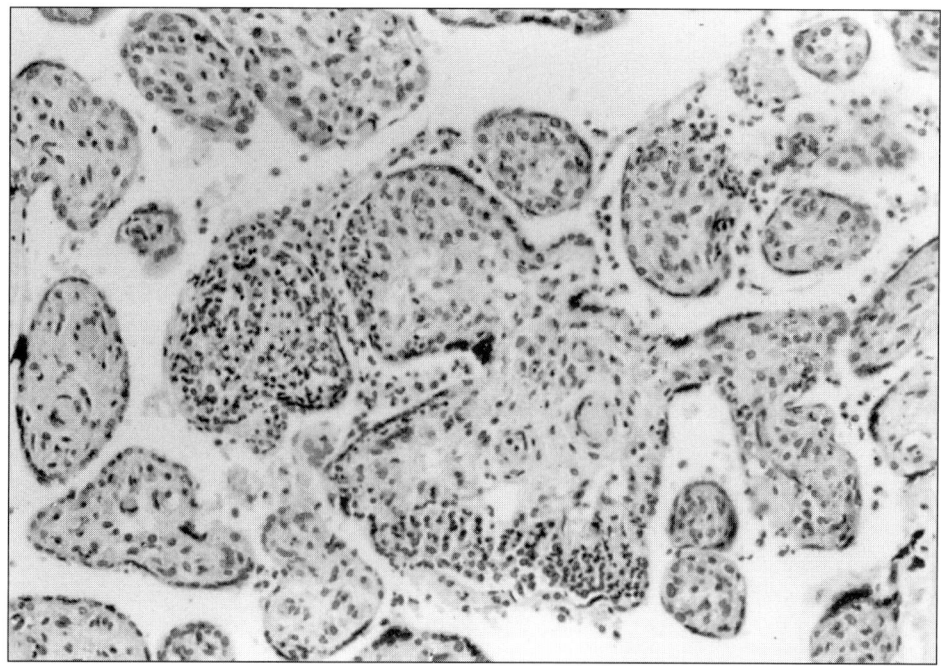

Figure 2–1. Acute villitis with villous microabscesses are scattered throughout the placenta. The fetus was infected with *L monocytogenes*.

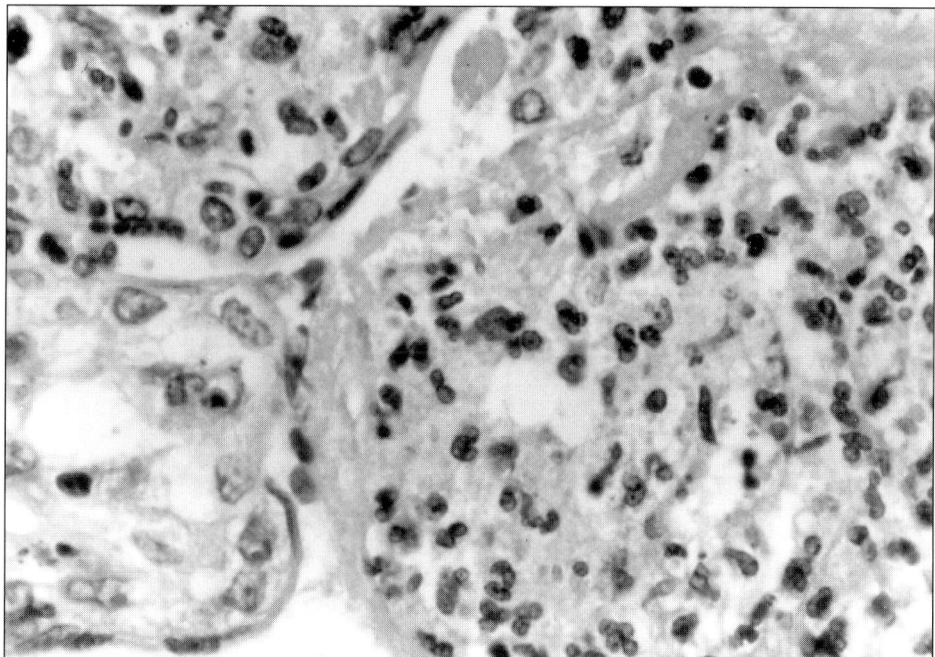

Figure 2–2. Necrosis of the villous stroma and trophoblast accompanies the acute inflammation.

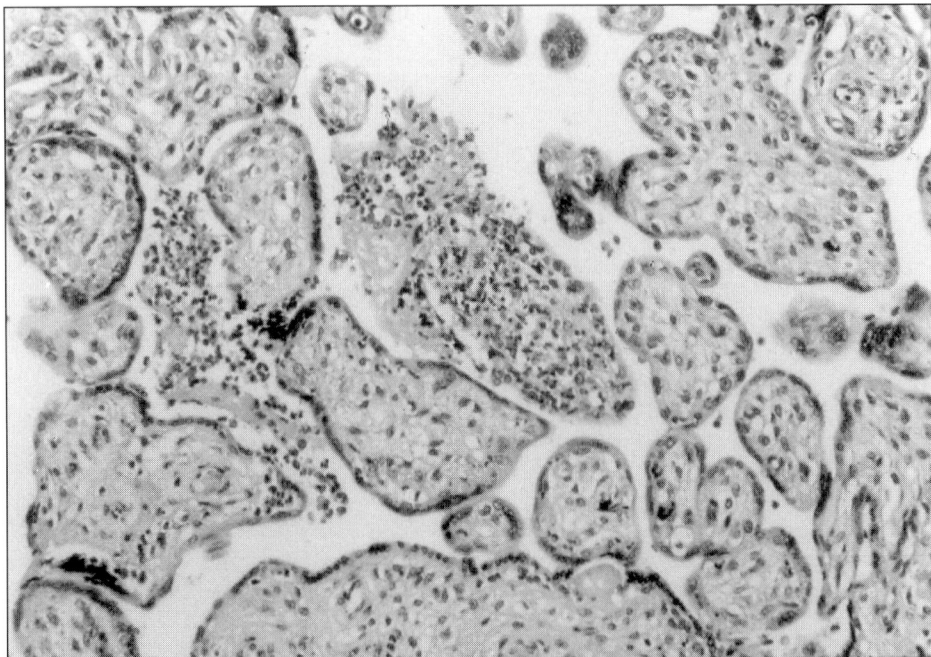

Figure 2-3. Acute villitis also occurs with fetal sepsis due to group B streptococcus (as shown here) and with other bacterial pathogens. The focal process is identical to that caused by *L monocytogenes*, but placental involvement is less extensive.

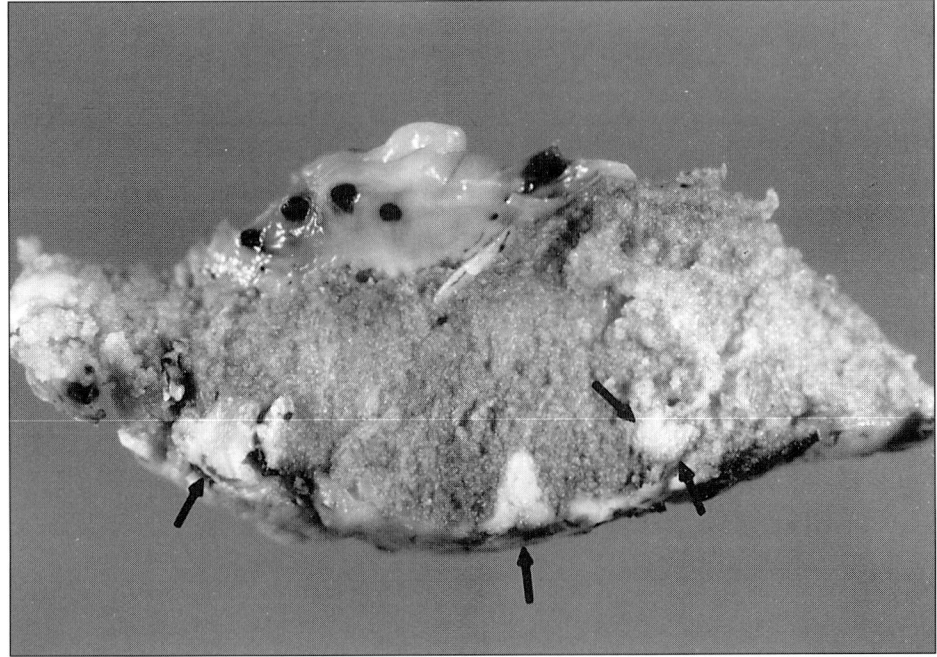

Figure 2-4. Macroabscesses (arrows) may be confused with infarcts. This is the placenta from the same case as shown in Figures 2-1 and 2-2.

perinatal or neonatal infections are divided into early onset infections (fetal infections or neonatal signs of disease in the first 3 to 5 days after birth) and late-onset infections.[10-12] Late-onset disease is often characterized by meningitis, beginning after 2 weeks of age. The meningitis may be granulomatous in long-standing cases. The interval between birth and signs of illness is usually longer with listeriosis than with late-onset neonatal infections with other organisms. Of the four common serotypes of *Listeria monocytogenes,* types I and IV account for 90% of the cases and type IV is most often implicated in neonatal meningitis.[13]

In fetal infections, the organism apparently invades the skin, producing a pustular rash. An alternative explanation for the rash is wide dissemination via the bloodstream of the fetus to the skin and other tissues. Miliary abscesses are widespread, as shown in the liver, adrenal gland, spleen, lung, and other organs. Mucosal necrosis is found in the gastrointestinal tract, and listeric organisms may be found in the edges of the lesions. The lungs usually are normal or have nonspecific pneumonitis or hemorrhage. The lesions in the liver and adrenal gland mimic the necrotic lesions of congenital herpes simplex infection, but the latter lesions do not have a neutrophilic response and cells have obvious intranuclear inclusions.[5,8] Listeric infection is yet another cause of hydrops fetalis.[14]

Infections with *L monocytogenes* are more common in Europe and other areas of the world than in the United States. In our institution, listeriosis accounted for only 3 cases among approximately 1,300 perinatal autopsies from 1981 to 1990. Nevertheless, in febrile pregnant women, listeria infection should be in the list of possible causes.[15] Transabdominal amniocentesis with Gram stain and culture has been used to establish the diagnosis.[16,17] In unexplained fetal deaths, cultures should be performed specifically to search for listeria.[18] Virulent listeria organisms are small gram-positive bacilli, similar to cocci, especially pneumococci. The organisms form palisades in tissues with X- and Y-shaped aggregates. At 20°C in liquid media, the bacteria have a tumbling motility. Virulent strains accounting for 96% of cases in the United States have serotypes 1/2a, 1/2b, and 4b.[19] Avirulent strains may be filamentous. Silver stains or Giemsa stains are more useful than Gram stain in demonstrating the organism in formalin-fixed tissues.

With a concerted effort to educate health care workers and food producers regarding the dangers of listeriosis, the incidence of perinatal cases in the United States decreased from 17.4 per 100,000 live births in 1989 to 8.6 per 100,000 live births in 1993 while the number of deaths was reduced from 481 in 1989 to 248 in 1993.[19]

DIAGNOSIS: Acute fetal listeriosis with diffuse acute villitis and miliary microabscesses throughout the body

References

1. Driscoll SG, Gorbach A, Feldman D. Congenital listeriosis: Diagnosis from placental studies. *Obstet Gynecol* 1962;20:216-220.
2. Yamazaki K, Price JT, Altshuler G. A placental view of the diagnosis and pathogenesis of congenital listeriosis. *Am J Obstet Gynecol* 1977;129:703-705.

3. Topalovski M, Yang SS, Boonpasat Y. Listeriosis of the placenta: Clinicopathologic study of seven cases. *Am J Obstet Gynecol* 1993;169:616-620.
4. Burn CG. Clinical and pathological features of an infection caused by a new pathogen of the genus *Listerella*. *Am J Pathol* 1936;12:341-348.
5. Vawter GF. Perinatal listeriosis. *Perspect Pediatr Pathol* 1981;6:153-166.
6. Fleming DW, Cochi SL, MacDonald KL, et al. Pasteurized milk as a vehicle of infection in an outbreak of listeriosis. *N Engl J Med* 1985;312:404-407.
7. Schuchat A, Lizano C, Boome CV, Swaminathan B, Kim C, Winn K. Outbreak of neonatal listeriosis associated with mineral oil. *Pediatr Infect Dis J* 1991;10:183-189.
8. Singer DB. Infections of fetuses and neonates. In: Wigglesworth JS, Singer DB, eds. *Textbook of Fetal and Perinatal Pathology*. Boston: Blackwell Scientific Publications; 1991:509.
9. Grieg A, Roth P. Colony-stimulating factor 1 in the human response to neonatal listeriosis. *Infection Immun* 1995;63:1595-1597.
10. Visintine A, Oleske JM, Nahmias AJ. *Listeria monocytogenes* infection in infants and children. *Am J Dis Child* 1977;131:393-397.
11. Bortolussi R. Perinatal infection due to *Listeria monocytogenes*. *Clin Invest Med* 1984;7:213-215.
12. Boucher M, Yonekura ML. Perinatal listeriosis (early-onset): Correlations of antenatal manifestations and neonatal outcome. *Obstet Gynecol* 1986;68:593-597.
13. Albritton WL, Wiggins GL, Feeley JC. Neonatal listeriosis: Distribution of serotypes in relation to age of onset of disease. *J Pediatr* 1976;88:481-483.
14. Gembruch U, Niesen M, Hansmann M, Knöpfle G. Listeriosis: A cause of non-immune hydrops fetalis. *Prenat Diagn* 1987;7:277-282.
15. Shirts SR, Brown MS, Bobbitt JR. Listeriosis and borreliosis as causes of antepartum fever. *Obstet Gynecol* 1983;62:256-261.
16. Petrilli ES, d'Ablanig G, Ledger WJ. *Listeria monocytogenes* chorioamnionitis: Diagnosis by transabdominal amniocentesis. *Obstet Gynecol* 1980;55:5s.
17. Mazor M, Froimovich M, Lazer S, Maymon E, Glezerman M. *Listeria monocytogenes:* The role of transabdominal amniocentesis in febrile patients with preterm labor. *Arch Gynecol Obstet* 1992;252:109-112.
18. Pitkin RM. Fetal death: Diagnosis and management. *Am J Obstet Gynecol* 1987;157:583-589.
19. Tappero JW, Schuchat A, Deaver KA, Mascola L, Wenger JD. Reduction in the incidence of human listeriosis in the United States: Effectiveness of prevention efforts? The Listeriosis Study Group. *JAMA* 1995;273:1118-1122.

Case Three

Contributed by Dan W. Hobohm, MD, and Dale Anne Singer, MD
Phoenix, Arizona

History

An 8-year-old Hispanic girl presented with bloody diarrhea. The patient underwent prior biopsies of the duodenum and stomach, specimens of which demonstrated *Helicobactor pylori* and lymphoid hyperplasia. There was a suspicion of small intestinal immunoproliferative disease and in the course of the clinical evaluation, a mass was detected in the jejunum. The patient also had splenomegaly, an elevated sedimentation rate, and microcytic hypochromic anemia resistant to iron therapy. Following the small bowel resection, the hemoglobin and sedimentation rate returned to normal. The patient is apparently well after 18 months.

Dr Dehner: A homogeneous gray-white mass measuring 5 to 6 cm in greatest dimension replaced the muscularis propria with a seemingly intact but flattened mucosa. The mass obliterated the anatomic markings of the bowel wall on cross section (Figure 3–1). Microscopically, there was transmural involvement by a fibroinflammatory process with effacement of the mucosa and replacement of the submucosa and muscularis propria (Figure 3–2). Residual mucosal glands and muscularis propria were identifiable in the midst of the spindle cells and collagen (Figure 3–3). There was a diffuse mixed inflammatory infiltrate of small lymphocytes and mature plasma cells interspersed among the spindle cells as either individual cells or small aggregates (Figure 3–4). Dense, hypocellular areas of collagen with an accompanying inflammatory infiltrate were present throughout the mass (see Figure 3–2). Foci of spindle cells were also prominent, and a storiform pattern was noted in the more extensive areas of spindle cells (Figure 3–5). The spindle cells displayed eosinophilic cytoplasm and a modest degree of nuclear atypism. Mitotic figures were noted, but they did not exceed two to three mitoses per 10 high-power fields. Atypical mitotic figures and necrosis were not evident.

The differential diagnosis of this stromal-mesenchymal and inflammatory mass of the jejunum includes a gastrointestinal stromal tumor, including a smooth muscle neoplasm (GIST); gastrointestinal autonomic neural tumor (GANT); and inflammatory myofibroblastic tumor (IMT).[1,2] On the basis of the light microscopic examination alone, these three tumor types may be difficult to discriminate from each other; however, there are some differences in the growth pattern and characteristics of the constituent cells (Table 3–1). Immunohistochemistry provides some assistance but is limited in terms of its ability to help discriminate between an IMT and a myogenic neoplasm. In our case, the

14   *Placental, Neonatal, and Pediatric Pathology*

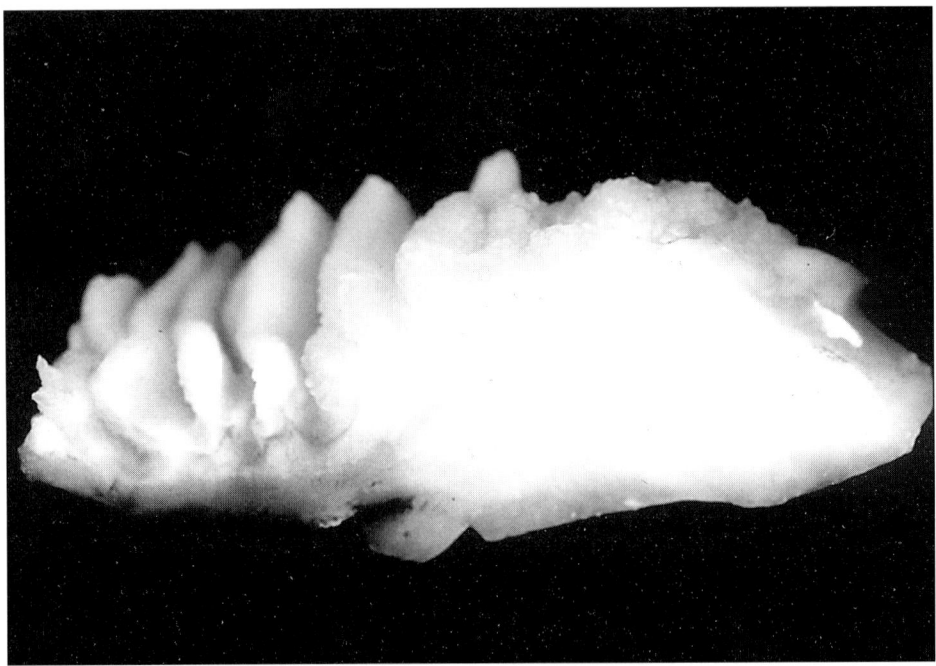

Figure 3–1. A cross section of the jejunum discloses a firm white mass filling and replacing the mucosa; a remnant of the muscularis mucosa is still identifiable.

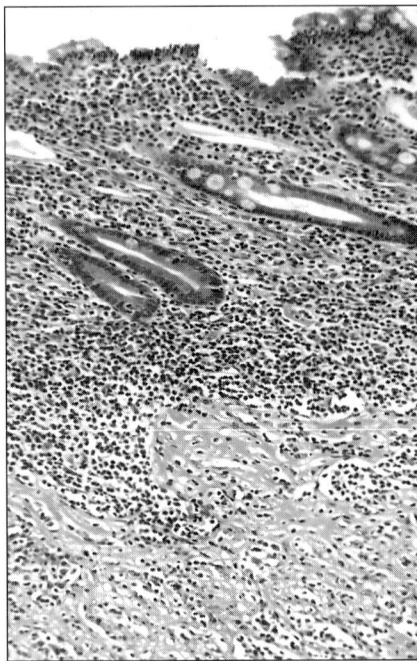

Figure 3–2. Mixed lymphocytic and plasmacellular infiltrate surrounds the mucosal glands. An accompanying focus of dense collagen is present in the submucosa.

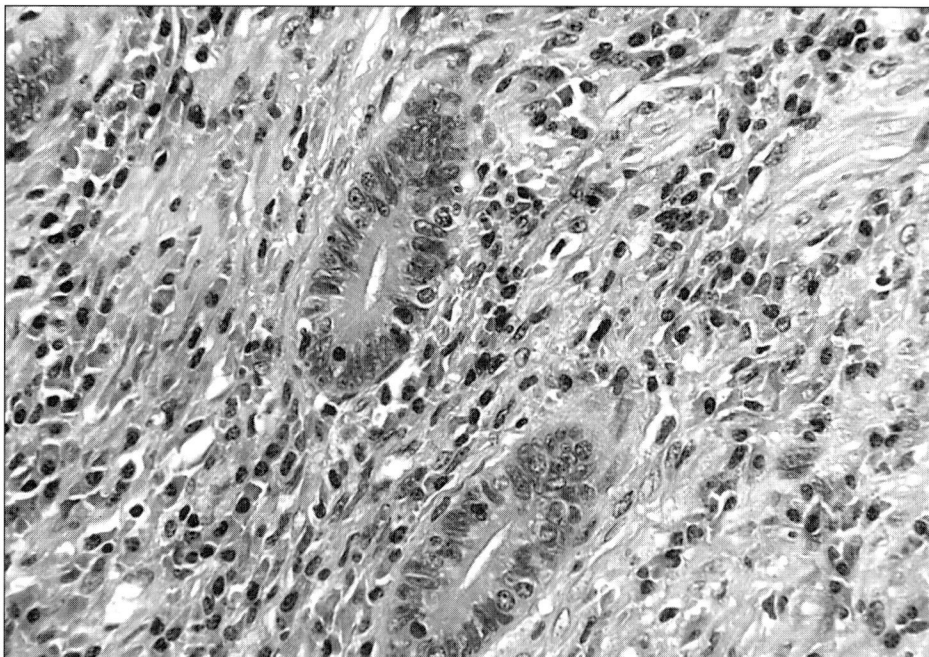

Figure 3–3. Spindle cells and mature plasma cells disrupt the architecture of the mucosa. The displacement of the intestinal glands is reminiscent of other infiltrative processes such as malignant lymphoma or Kaposi's sarcoma.

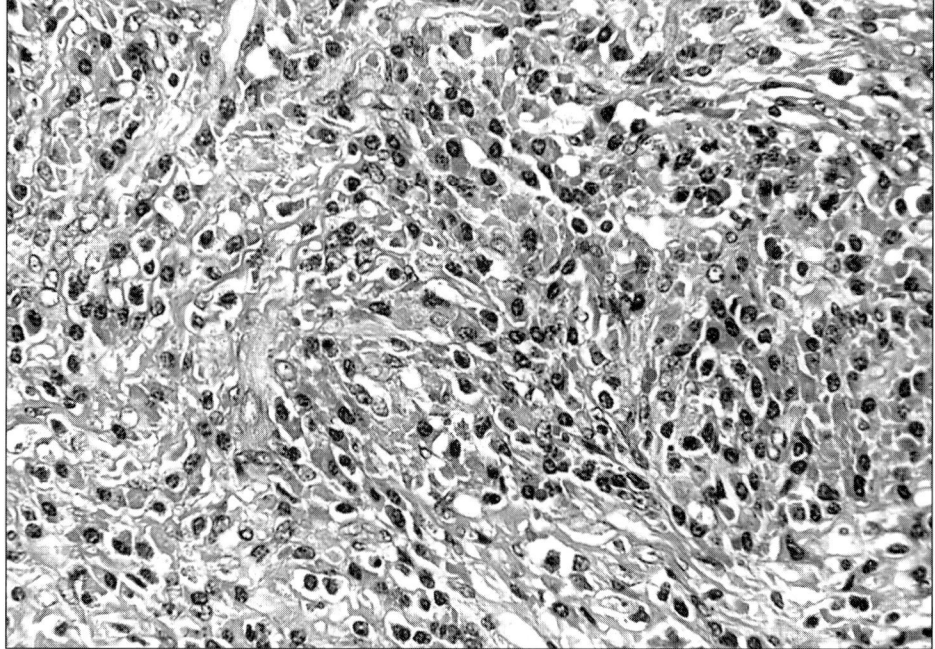

Figure 3–4. Plasma cells are evenly distributed in a background of spindle cells, which are partially obscured by the dense infiltrate.

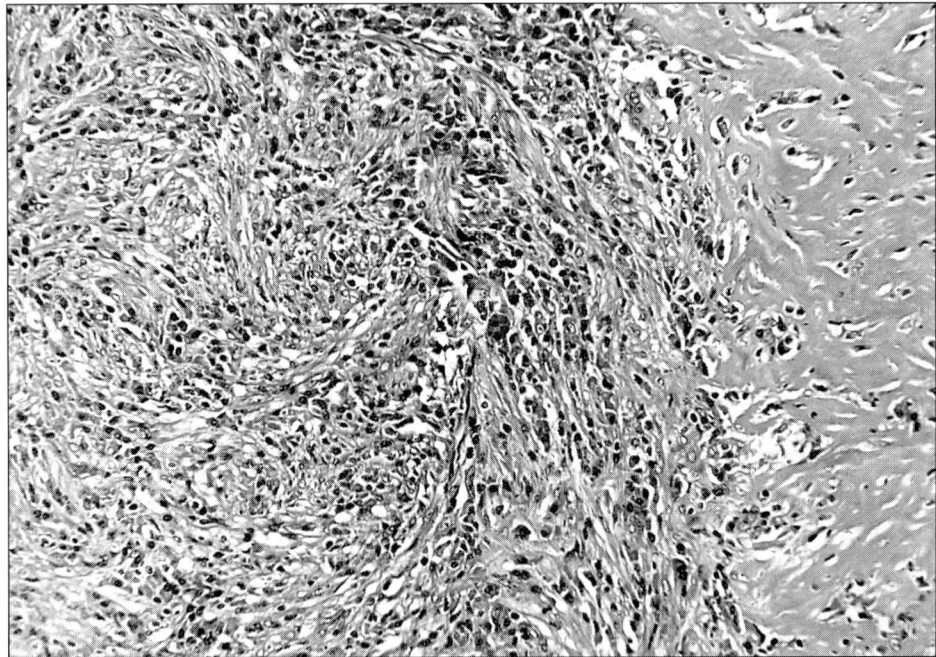

Figure 3–5. The spindle cell component with its storiform pattern is abruptly replaced by dense, hyalinized collagen.

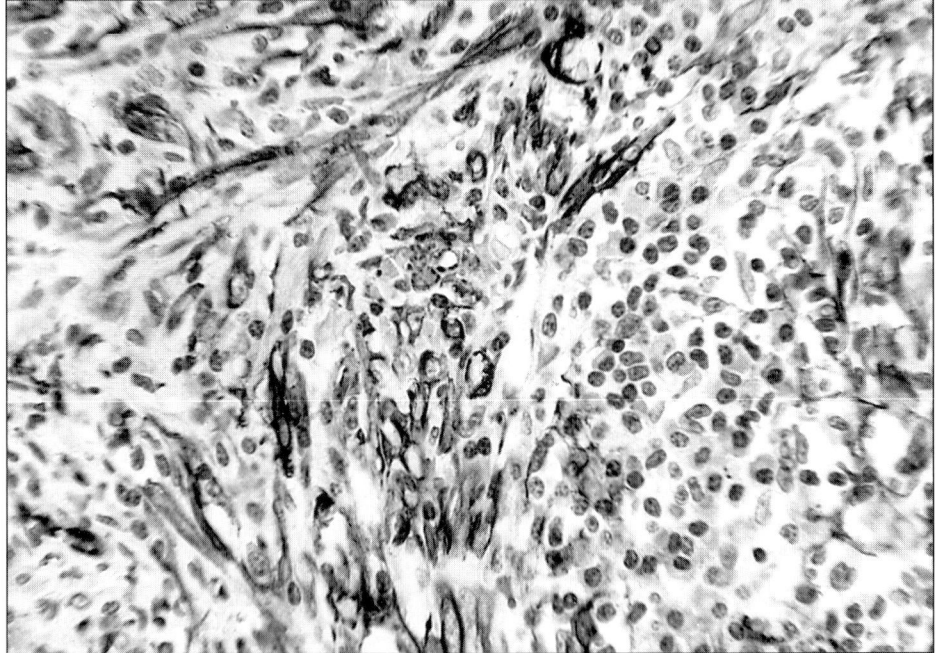

Figure 3–6. The spindle cells are intensely immunoreactive for smooth muscle actin.

Table 3–1. Pathologic and Immunohistochemical Features of Intestinal Stromal-Mesenchymal Tumors

	Sites	Histologic features	Immunophenotype
IMT	Small intestine/ mesentery	Mixture of spindle cells with storiform or inter-fascicular pattern, cellular-myxoid pattern, dense collagen, plasma cells and lymphocytes	VMA SMA MSA
GIST	Small intestine/ stomach	Spindle and epithelioid cells, occasional nuclear palisading, nodular or multinotdular growth, replacement rather than overgrowth of bowel wall	VIM SMA DES S-100
GANT	Small intestine/ mesentery	Variable, but plump, spindle cells and/or epithelioid cells, interfascicular or diffuse patterns	VIM NSE SYN S-100

Abbreviations: IMT = inflammatory myofibroblastic tumor; GIST = gastrointestinal stromal tumor; GANT = gastrointestinal autonomic neural tumor; VMA = vanillylmandelic acid; VIM = vimentin; SMA = smooth muscle actin; MSA = muscle-specific actin; S-100 = S-100 protein; DES = desmin; NSE = neuron-specific enolase; SYN = synaptophysin.

spindle cells showed diffuse and intense immunoreactivity for vimentin and smooth muscle actin, and there was focal, less intense positivity for muscle-specific actin (HHF-35) and desmin (Figure 3–6). The blood vessels in the background served as internal controls for the latter two antibodies. Neuron-specific enolase, Leu 7, S-100 protein, cytokeratin, and synaptophysin were all nonreactive. The plasma cells are polyclonal for κ and λ light chains.

Since the immunophenotype of the spindle cells indicated that they were myogenic, the diagnosis would appear to be a smooth muscle neoplasm. However, the myofibroblast is also characterized by its myogenic phenotype.[3] The two morphologic attributes of this tumor that were regarded as central to the differentiation between a myogenic neoplasm and a myofibroblastic proliferation were the inhomogeneous pattern and prominent inflammatory component anticipated in an IMT. Most stromal neoplasms of the gastrointestinal tract have a circumscribed and/or multinodular growth in the muscularis and some variation in histologic findings, such as more or less uniform spindle cells and/or epithelioid cells without an appreciable inflammatory component except for neutrophils and histiocytes in and around areas of necrosis. The tumor cells in a GIST may be arranged in cords, trabeculae, and Verocay body–like structures producing a neural or neuroendocrine-like appearance. Some stromal neoplasms may have features of a classic smooth muscle tumor yet are devoid of any myogenic markers. Our case was characterized by an infiltrative growth with the obliteration or entrapment of residual normal structures of the jejunum, whereas most myogenic tumors of the intestinal tract have pushing borders with an intact muscularis at the periphery of the circumscribed mass or nodules. The overlying mucosa may be focally ulcerated, but is otherwise well preserved in most GISTs. The predominant pattern of vimentin and smooth muscle actin immunoreactivity of an IMT is characteristic of the type of myofibroblasts that are seen in infantile myofibromatosis.

IMT is the proposed designation by the World Health Organization for the tumefactive process that has been known for many years as inflammatory pseudotumor, plasma cell granuloma, and xanthomatous postinflammatory pseudotumor at a time when this tumefaction was recognized almost exclusively in the lung.[4-8] However, this same entity has been reported in virtually every anatomic site and organ that one may select at random including the skin, brain, spleen, lymph node, heart, and bladder.[9-11] More recently, the IMT has been reported in the abdominal cavity as inflammatory fibrosarcoma.[12] Given the plethora of designations, many of which we have not listed, it is not surprising that different conclusions have been reached about the nosology and etiology of the IMT.

The two most common anatomic sites of IMT are the lung and mesentery-omentum with or without involvement of the contiguous small intestine, usually in the region of the distal small intestine.[13] Regardless of anatomic site, the majority of patients are less than 20 years old at diagnosis. In our series of 84 extrapulmonary IMTs, the mean age was almost 10 years and the youngest case occurred in a 3-month-old infant.[14] Most patients present with a mass and abdominal pain, but a minority of patients also have fever (weeks' to months' duration), failure to thrive (especially prominent in the younger patients), anemia (hypochromic microcytic anemia with normal serum iron), polyclonal hypergammaglobulinemia, elevated sedimentation rate, thrombocytosis, and plasmacytosis of the bone marrow. Our patient had anemia and an elevated sedimentation rate, but did not have immunoglobulin abnormalities. Once the mass has been excised, the constitutional manifestations, if present, typically disappear over days or weeks as in our case. Clinical and laboratory abnormalities have been known to reappear in those few patients in whom additional IMTs develop after an initial resection. To date, the cause of the IMT is unknown, but it would appear that cytokines, particularly IL-1 and/or IL-6, produced by the tumor mediate many of the constitutional signs and symptoms.[15] In the lung, it has been proposed that the IMT is a manifestation of unresolved pneumonia in some cases.[16] The possible role of Epstein-Barr virus has also been explored without conclusive results.

The IMT, as in our case, typically has a variable microscopic appearance that may be appreciated in the gross examination. Dystrophic calcification and even metaplastic bone are present in a minority of cases.[17] Whether the mass is in the lung or mesentery, it is usually well circumscribed, but nonencapsulated. Multifocal masses in the abdominal cavity or a separate mass in the lung and brain in the same patient have raised questions about the capacity for the IMT to metastasize.[18] These distinct masses are probably no more metastatic in nature than the multifocal lesions of fibromatosis or myofibromatosis. Histologically, an IMT may resemble nodular fasciitis, fibrous histiocytoma with its storiform pattern, fibromatosis, and sclerosing mediastinitis or mesenteritis with its dense collagenous stroma. Sclerosing mesenteritis is a diffuse process rather than a discrete mass like most IMTs. On a histologic basis alone, it may be difficult to differentiate an IMT from sclerosing mesenteritis simply on the basis of isolated microscopic fields.[19] Rarely, IMT may undergo malignant transformation to a high-grade mononuclear cell neoplasm with the immunophenotype of macrophages or histiocytes.[14] We have also had the experience of post-transplant lymphoproliferative disorder developing in two children after hepatic transplantation for IMT of the liver.

What is the IMT? Is it an exuberant reaction to a prior undocumented infection or a bona fide neoplastic process? A few cases in children have been accompanied by nodal changes resembling Castleman's disease. There are isolated reports of cytogenetic abnormalities; a translocation, t(2;9)(q1,3;p2,2), was detected in a jejunal IMT from a 3-year-old boy, and a ringed supernumerary chromosome, 47XX+r, has been identified in an IMT of the lung in a 5-year-old girl.[20,21] If indeed the IMT is a clonal proliferation, then it probably should be regarded as a neoplasm. The IMT is capable of locally aggressive behavior, especially in the case of hepatic and pulmonary IMTs, which may grow into blood vessels.[22,23] There is no question that the IMT may progress to an overtly malignant process, which is recognized by a round cell proliferation with histiocytic features.[14] However, we do not believe that the IMT should be regarded as malignant from its inception, which is implied by the designation of *inflammatory fibrosarcoma*.[12] Most patients in our experience do well after surgical resection, as seems to be the case in our patient.[14]

DIAGNOSIS: Inflammatory myofibroblastic tumor of the jejunum

References

1. Franquemont DW, Frierson HF Jr. Muscle differentiation and clinicopathologic features of gastrointestinal stromal tumors. *Am J Surg Pathol* 1992;16: 947-954.
2. Lauwers GY, Erlandson RA, Casper ES, Brennan MF, Woodruff JM. Gastrointestinal autonomic nerve tumors: A clinicopathological, immunohistochemical, and ultrastructural study of 12 cases. *Am J Surg Pathol* 1993; 17:887-897.
3. Schurch W, Seemayer TA, Gabbiani G. Myofibroblasts. In: Sternberg SS, ed. *Histology for Pathologists*. New York: Raven Press, Ltd; 1992:109-144.
4. Weiss SW. *Histologic Typing of Soft Tissue Tumors*. 2nd ed. Berlin: Springer-Verlag; 1994:48.
5. Bahadori M, Liebow AA. Plasma cell granulomas of the lung. *Cancer* 1973;31: 191-208.
6. Pearl M, Woolley MM. Pulmonary xanthomatous postinflammatory pseudotumor in children. *J Pediatr Surg* 1973;8:255-261.
7. Titus JL, Harrison EG, Clagett OT, et al. Xanthomatous and inflammatory pseudotumors of the lung. *Cancer* 1962;15:522-538.

8. Pettinato G, Manivel JC, DeRosa N, Dehner LP. Inflammatory myofibroblastic tumor plasma cell granuloma: Clinicopathologic study of 20 cases with immunohistochemical and ultrastructural observations. *Am J Clin Pathol* 1990;94:538-546.
9. Hurt MA, Santa Cruz DJ. Cutaneous inflammatory pseudotumor: Lesions resembling "inflammatory pseudotumor" or "plasma cell granulomas" of extracutaneous sites. *Am J Surg Pathol* 1990; 14:764-773.
10. Thomas RM, Jaffe ES, Zarate-Osorno A, Medeiros LJ. Inflammatory pseudotumor of the spleen: A clinicopathologic and immunophenotypic study of eight cases. *Arch Pathol Lab Med* 1993; 117:921-926.
11. Albores-Saavedra J, Manivel JC, Essenfeld H, et al. Pseudosarcomatous myofibroblastic proliferations in the urinary bladder of children. *Cancer* 1990;66:1234-1241.
12. Meis JM, Enzinger FM. Inflammatory fibrosarcoma of the mesentery and retroperitoneum: A tumor closely simulating inflammatory pseudotumor. *Am J Surg Pathol* 1991;15:1146-1156.
13. Anthony PP. Inflammatory pseudotumor (plasma cell granuloma) of lung, liver and other organs. *Histopathology* 1993;23:501-503.
14. Coffin CM, Watterson J, Priest JR, Dehner LP. Extrapulmonary inflammatory myofibroblastic tumor (inflammatory pseudotumor): A clinicopathologic and immunohistochemical study of 84 cases. *Am J Surg Pathol* 1995;19:859-872.
15. Rohrlich P, Peuchmaur M, Cocci SN, et al. Interleukin-6 and interleukin-1b production in a pediatric plasma cell granuloma. *Am J Surg Pathol* 1995;19: 590-595.
16. Matsubara D, Tan-Liu NS, Kenney RM, Mark EJ. Inflammatory pseudotumor of the lung: Progression from organizing pneumonia to fibrous histiocytoma or to plasma cell granuloma in 32 cases. *Hum Pathol* 1988;19: 807-814.
17. Vujanic GM, Berry PJ, Frank JD. Inflammatory pseudotumor of the kidney with extensive metaplastic bone. *Pediatr Pathol* 1992;12:557-561.
18. Chan YF, White J, Brash H. Metachronous pulmonary and cerebral inflammatory pseudotumors in a child. *Pediatr Pathol* 1994;14:805-815.
19. Kelly JK, Hwang WS. Idiopathic retractile (sclerosing) mesenteritis and its differential diagnosis. *Am J Surg Pathol* 1989;13:513-521.
20. Treissman SP, Gillis A, Lee CLY, et al. Omental-mesenteric inflammatory pseudotumor: Cytogenetic demonstration of genetic changes and monoclonality in one tumor. *Cancer* 1994;73:1433-1437.
21. Su L, Sheldon S, Weiss SW. Inflammatory myofibroblastic tumor: Cytogenetic evidence supporting clonal orgin. *Mod Pathol* 1995;8:12A. Abstract.
22. Broughan TA, Fischer WL, Tuthill RJ. Vascular invasion by hepatic inflammatory pseudotumor: A clinicopathologic study. *Cancer* 1993;71:2934-2940.
23. Warter A, Satge D, Roeslin N. Angioinvasive plasma cell granulomas of the lung. *Cancer* 1987;59:435-443.

Case Four

Contributed by Frederic B. Askin, MD
Baltimore, Maryland

History

This 1-year-old female infant presented with a tumor on the back that had been present for an undetermined period but had recently increased in size. A firm mass measuring 10 × 4 cm was palpable in the subcutis. A wide local excision was performed. The patient has not experienced an interval recurrence since the surgery of 1 year ago.

Dr Dehner: A generous excision of the mass on the back of this infant yielded a firm, indurated, pale tan tumor measuring 10 × 4 cm. The overlying ellipse of skin was also indurated and there was apparent involvement of the dermis by the underlying process, whose major component was centered in the subcutis. Sections of the tumor revealed a spindle cell proliferation in the subcutaneous tissues with apparent noncircumscribed growth, as represented by the presence of small stromal nodules, and bands and bundles of spindle cells randomly distributed throughout the adipose tissue (Figure 4–1). Focally, the fat had some immature features to be anticipated in an infant of this age. There was nothing to suggest the presence of a lipoblastoma. Rather, the microscopic features of small, somewhat immature "neuroid" bundles and fibrous bands, some of which had accompanying immature or maturing bundles at the periphery or were seemingly incorporated into the fibrous strands, are characteristic of the fibrous hamartoma of infancy (FHI) (Figure 4–2). In some areas of the tumor, it was possible to follow the spindle cells into the dermis mainly along the connective tissue planes surrounding the hair follicles (Figure 4–3). This feature of FHI may allow for the diagnosis to be made or suggested from a full-thickness biopsy specimen of skin. However, most cases, as in this infant, are diagnosed on the basis of deep excisional biopsy results.

Immunohistochemistry disclosed that the more obviously fibrous areas yielded a strong reaction for vimentin and smooth muscle actin, whereas the immature nodules were weakly reactive for vimentin but were nonreactive for smooth muscle actin (Figure 4–4).

Fibrous hamartoma of infancy (FHI) is one in a group of fibrous or myofibroblastic proliferative disorders that occur exclusively or almost so in children (Table 4–1).[1,2] However, FHI was one of the least common fibrous tumors of childhood in our series, as evidenced by the fact that only 5% of cases were FHI compared to infantile myofibromatosis, which represented over 20% of cases in the same series.[3]

22 *Placental, Neonatal, and Pediatric Pathology*

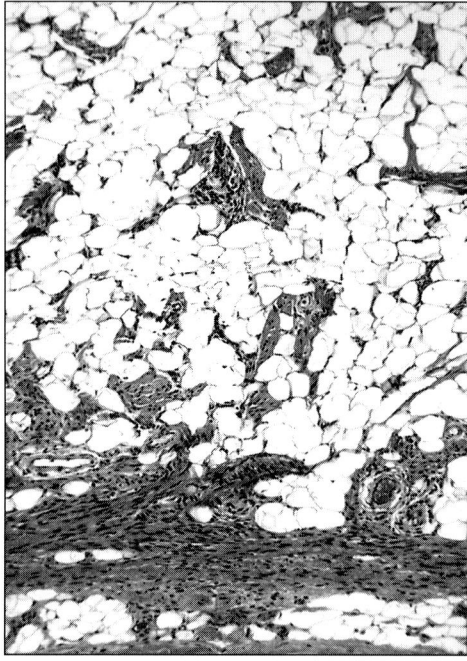

Figure 4–1. Multiple distinct islands of mesenchymal tissue are distributed randomly in the subcutaneous fat. Growth along or into the deep fascia is a common finding in fibrous hamartomas of infancy.

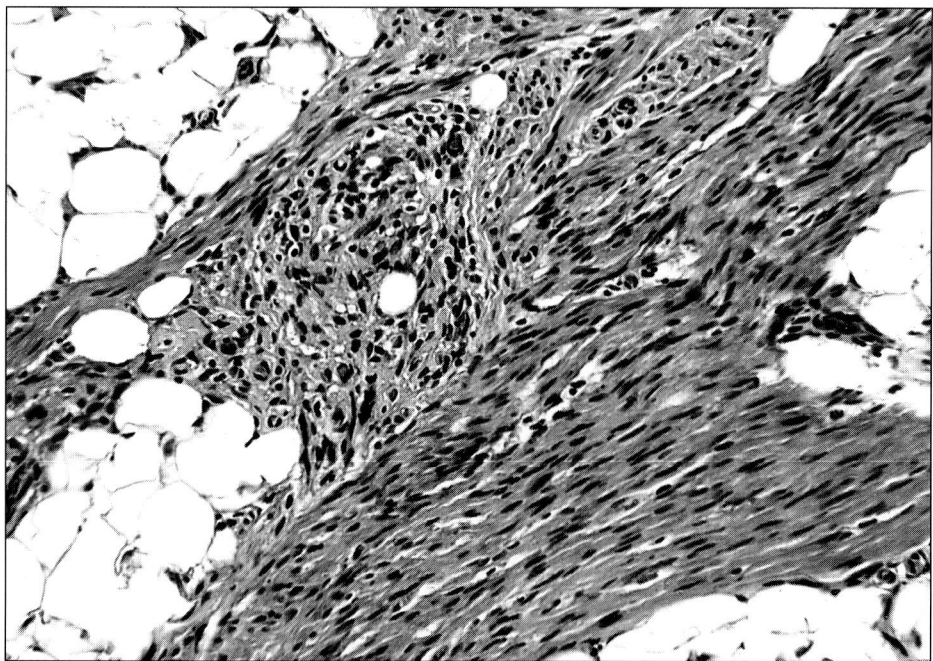

Figure 4–2. A so-called neuroid bundle or nodule representing immature stromal cells is recognized by its relatively dense cellularity, ovoid hyperchromatic nuclei, and location at the periphery of the mature fibroblasts or myofibroblasts.

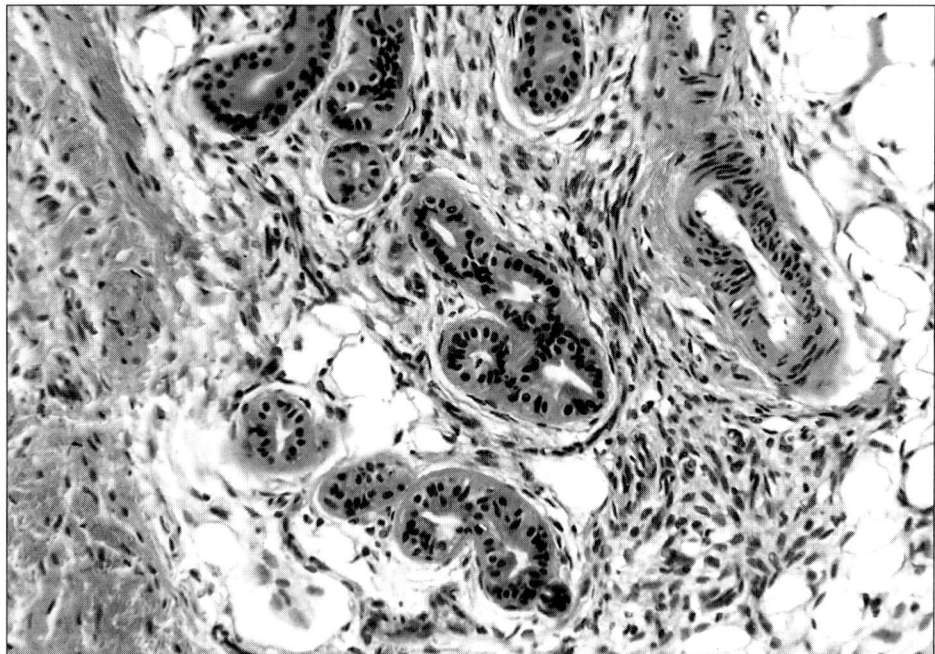

Figure 4–3. Immature stromal cells have extended around sweat glands in the deep dermis. This pattern of dermal involvement contrasts with the multiple circumscribed nodules present throughout the dermis in infantile myofibromatosis and the diffuse overgrowth of the dermis and subcutis of infantile digital fibromatosis.

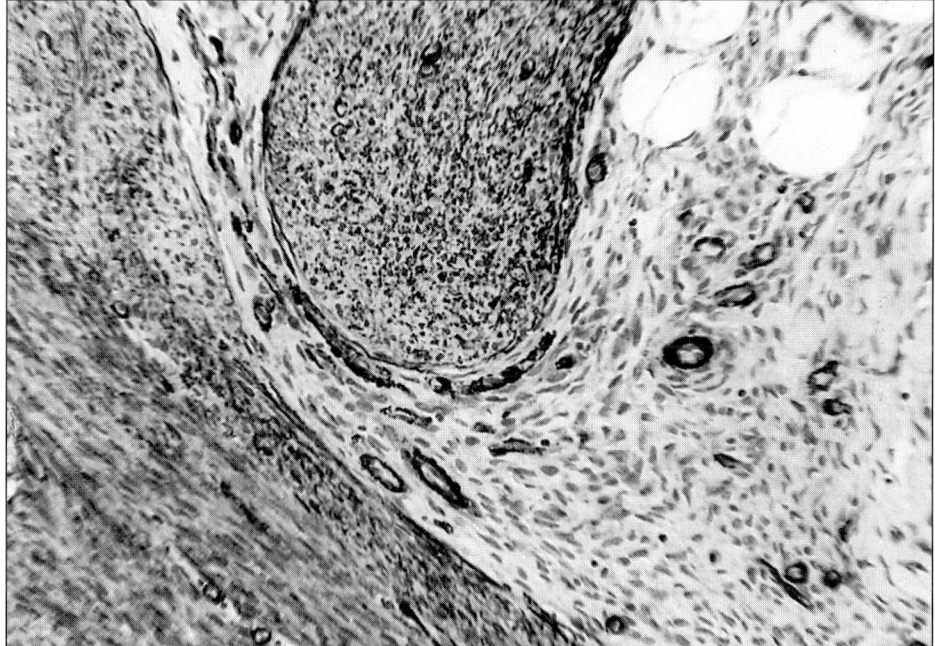

Figure 4–4. The immature stroma is nonreactive for smooth muscle actin, in contrast to the intense immunopositivity in the mature fibroblasts and myofibroblasts.

Table 4–1. Myofibroblastic Proliferations of Childhood

Nodular fasciitis
Cranial fasciitis
Inflammatory myofibroblastic tumor
Calcifying fibrous pseudotumor
Infantile myofibromatosis
Composite myofibromatosis
Infantile fibromatosis
Fibrous hamartoma of infancy
Digital fibromatosis
Fibromatosis colli
Hyalin fibromatosis
Calcifying aponeurotic fibroma

Reye in 1956 reported his experience with six cases of "certain subdermal fibromatous tumors of infancy," first noted in each case before 1 year of age.[4] Two tumors were noted at birth. The anatomic distribution of these six tumors was the following: axilla (2), retroauricular (1), posterior neck (1), chest wall (1), and groin (1). Following this initial report, Enzinger in 1965[5] described his experience with 30 cases, which remained the largest published series until the study of Sotelo-Avila and Bale.[6] The latter report is interesting because many of the cases had been reviewed by Reye during his many years at the Royal Alexandra Hospital for Children in Sydney, Australia. The mean age at diagnosis in the latter series was 16 months. With the exception of a 4-year-old child, virtually all cases have been diagnosed at or before 30 months of age. There is a distinct male predilection (70% to 75% of cases) and a preference for the upper and lower trunk, so that our case is a typical one except for the fact that the patient is a female. A mass noted at birth is recorded in approximately 15% of cases. It has been our experience that the FHI may present in sites other than the usual ones.[7] In addition to the head and neck and extremities, FHI has a tendency to occur in the region of the groin and scrotum, which has been reported in a series by Popek et al.[8] Most FHIs generally do not exceed 3 to 5 cm in greatest dimension, so that our case is one of the largest examples that I have personally seen. There is one report of multiple lesions, which is highly unusual.[9] Excision is curative in 85% to 90% of cases with a local recurrence rate of 10% to 15%.[10-13] When an FHI recurs, it may be difficult to appreciate the characteristic microscopic features that have been replaced by a fibrous proliferation resembling a common desmoid tumor.

Various studies in the past have confirmed that the FHI is a myofibroblastic proliferation as demonstrated by electron microscopy and immunohistochemistry.[14-16] Most standard classifications include the FHI as a "benign fibrous tumor" or a "fibrous tumor of infancy and childhood."[17] Its hamartomatous nature is seriously questioned. One reason for regarding the FHI as a hamartoma is related to the presence of fat with immature features, but lipoblastic-appearing fat is the norm in the subcutaneous tissues of an infant. Unlike a true hamartoma, FHI is a process with the potential to recur.

An interesting aspect of the FHI is its apparent ability to undergo maturation. The presence and number of immature neuroid bundles tend to vary from one tumor to another—these bundles or nodules are seemingly incorporated and overgrown by the more mature fibrous or desmoid-like tissue. This process is not necessarily correlated with the age of the patient at the time of excision.

DIAGNOSIS: Fibrous hamartoma of infancy

References

1. Enzinger FM, Weiss SW. *Soft Tissue Tumors*. 3rd ed. St. Louis: Mosby; 1995: 231-236.
2. Cooper PH. Fibrous proliferations of infancy and childhood. *J Cutan Pathol* 1992;19:257-267.
3. Coffin CM, Dehner LP. Fibroblastic-myofibroblastic tumors in children and adolescents: A clinicopathologic study of 108 examples in 103 patients. *Pediatr Pathol* 1991;11:559-588.
4. Reye RDK. A consideration of certain subdermal 'fibromatous tumors' of infancy. *J Pathol Bacteriol* 1956; 72:149-154.
5. Enzinger FM. Fibrous hamartoma of infancy. *Cancer* 1965;18:241-248.
6. Sotelo-Avila C, Bale PM. Subdermal fibrous hamartoma of infancy: Pathology of 40 cases and differential diagnosis. *Pediatr Pathol* 1994;14:39-52.
7. Kirby W, Coffin CM, Dehner LP. Fibrous hamartoma of infancy: A clinicopathologic study of 19 cases emphasizing unusual sites and an expanded age range. *Pediatr Pathol* 1994;14:547-548.
8. Popek EJ, Montgomery EA, Fourcroy JL. Fibrous hamartoma of infancy in the genital region: Findings in 15 cases. *J Urol* 1994;152:990-993.
9. Jung PM, Hong EK. Fibrous hamartoma of infancy manifested as multiple nodules: A case report. *J Korean Med Sci* 1990;5:243-247.
10. Paller AS, Gonzalez-Crussi F, Sherman JO. Fibrous hamartoma of infancy: Eight additional cases and a review of the literature. *Arch Dermatol* 1989;125:88-91.
11. Efem SE, Ekpo MD. Clinicopathologic features of untreated fibrous hamartoma of infancy. *J Clin Pathol* 1993;46:522-524.
12. Loyer EM, Shabb NS, Mahon TG, Eftekhari F. Fibrous hamartoma of infancy: MR-pathologic correlation. *J Comput Assist Tomogr* 1992;16:311-313.
13. Lee JT, Girvan DP, Armstrong RF. Fibrous hamartoma of infancy. *J Pediatr Surg* 1988;23:759-761.
14. Groisman G, Lichtig C. Fibrous hamartoma of infancy: An immunohistochemical and ultrastructural study. *Hum Pathol* 1991;22:914-918.
15. Michal M, Mukenshabl P, Chlumska A, Kodet R. Fibrous hamartoma of infancy: A study of eight cases with immunohistochemical and electron microscopic findings. *Pathol Res Pract* 1992;188:1049-1053.
16. Fletcher CDM, Powell G, Van Noorden S, McKee PH. Fibrous hamartoma of infancy: A histochemical and immunohistochemical study. *Histopathology* 1988;12:65-74.
17. Weiss SW. *Histological Typing of Soft Tissue Tumors*. 2nd ed. Berlin: Springer-Verlag; 1994:15-19.

Case Five

Contributed by Don B. Singer, MD
Providence, Rhode Island

History

This male fetus was stillborn at 21 to 22 weeks' gestation. The mother was 28 years old and in her fifth pregnancy. Premature rupture of membranes had occurred 3 weeks previously. She had no additional signs or symptoms other than minimal vaginal bleeding. Spontaneous labor began, and despite attempts to stop the contractions, she delivered the fetus 3 days later.

Dr Singer: The sections are of liver with extensive extramedullary hematopoiesis in the sinusoids and in the portal connective tissues (Figure 5–1). On close inspection, the elements in the sinusoids have mostly round nuclei, but in every field bean-shaped nuclei or band forms are found. The nuclei, whether rounded or grooved, are larger than those of erythropoiesis and have prominent chromatin granules and sharply defined nuclear borders (Figure 5–2). Cytoplasmic granules are present in some of these cells. The granules are amphophilic, and some are distinctly eosinophilic. Large numbers of nucleated erythroid precursors are also present in the sinusoids. They appear in clusters and have smaller nuclei with orange cytoplasm. The more mature erythroid nuclei are solid with dense dark blue-black chromatin. Megakaryocytes are present, if at all, in very small numbers. The portal tracts have a mixture of hematopoietic cells similar to those in the sinusoids, but these are predominantly granulocytes. Especially easily identified are those with eosinophilic granules in the cytoplasm. Erythroid cells are sparse in the portal areas. Stains for granulocyte granules are strongly positive.

Other changes in the fetus are petechiae in the thymus, pleura, pericardium, and adrenal gland, and subcapsular hemorrhage in the liver (Figure 5–1). Germinal matrix hemorrhages are found in the brain. The placenta shows acute diffuse severe chorioamnionitis and umbilical vasculitis involving all three vessels. *Xanthomonas maltophilia* was cultured from the heart's blood. Incidental lesions were postaxial polydactyly of the left hand and mild varus deformity of the right foot. Chromosome analysis demonstrated a male karyotype, 46, XY.

Fetuses and liveborn babies in the second trimester of gestation have abundant hematopoiesis in the liver. The liver is the main source of both red blood cells and white blood cells for the fetus until after 30 weeks' gestation while the bone marrow gradually assumes its role as the primary producer of blood cells. In most fetuses and babies at 20 to 23 weeks' gestation, the hepatic sinusoids serve as the reservoir and incubator for large numbers of erythroid precursors, the nucleated red blood cells. Normocytes and earlier erythroid forms occupy as much as 15% to 20% of the parenchyma at this stage of gestation. As time goes

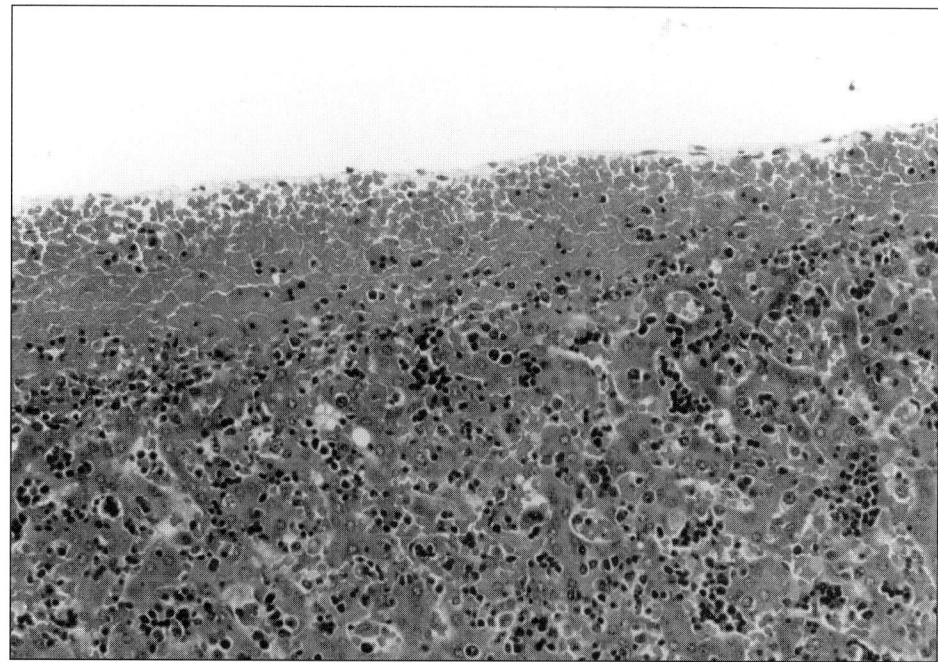

Figure 5–1. The liver sinusoids are packed with hematopoietic cells. Both erythroid and granulocytic series are represented. A subcapsular hemorrhage is present at the surface (the capsular collagenous tissue is artifactually absent).

on, the proportion of nucleated erythroids gradually falls to less than 1% of the hepatic parenchyma, the expected proportion by 40 weeks of intrauterine life.[1] In this case the cells are larger than erythroid precursors. They are granulocyte precursors and this line of hematopoietic cells should predominate in the portal connective tissue, not the hepatic sinusoids. Many of these cells are identified by their large eosinophilic granules. Eosinophils normally account for 10% to 20% of granulocytes in premature infants. In the second trimester, fetuses may have absolute eosinophil counts of $1.5 \times 10^9/L$ to $3.0 \times 10^9/L$, representing up to one-third of total granulocytes in the first month of life in premature infants.[2,3] Other causes of eosinophilia are Rh disease, total parenteral nutrition, and transfusions. IgE is not increased in these cases.[4]

Excessive granulopoiesis in fetuses or newborn infants can be caused by infection, stress, or asphyxia. It is usually mild in all three of these situations, but with some infections, granulopoiesis can manifest to this degree in the hepatic sinusoids. Stallmach and Karolyi found that hepatic granulopoiesis is increased as much as 12-fold in cases of fetal infection.[5] Chorioamnionitis and funisitis are present in virtually all such cases. The demonstration of the true nature of the hematopoietic cells may require special stains, such as the Leder stain for granules, lysozyme stains, or leukocyte common antigen (LCA). These test results were positive in our case.

28   Placental, Neonatal, and Pediatric Pathology

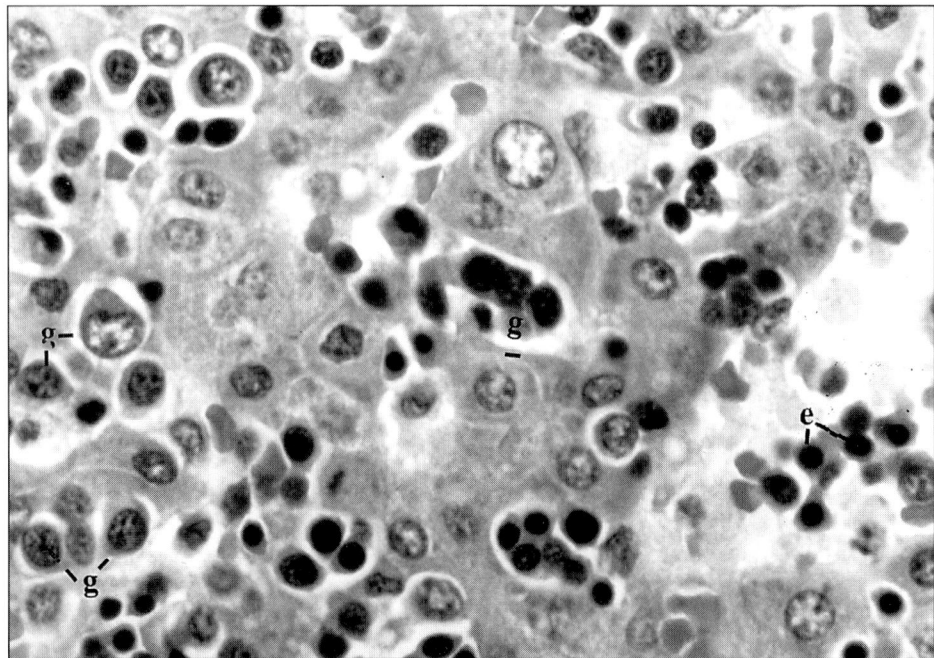

Figure 5–2. Sinusoidal hematopoiesis is prominent. Erythroid precursors (*e*) have homogeneous dark nuclei centrally placed in the cytoplasm. Granulocytic precursors (*g*) are large with vesicular nuclei and coarse chromatin granules.

Myeloproliferative syndromes, myelodysplastic syndromes, and congenital leukemias must also be considered. Congenital leukemia is a rare disorder, encountered only once in our institution in the last 105,000 births. It is usually a nonlymphocytic type, in contrast to leukemia in older children. Many congenital leukemias are monocytic, myelomonocytic, and megakaryoblastic, the latter found especially in cases of trisomy 21.[6] Congenital leukemia has been diagnosed only rarely in premature infants and stillborns.[7,8] Hydrops and infiltration of several tissues by blasts were features in these cases but were not found in our case.

Myeloproliferative disorders as they are known in adults are rare in children[9] and evidently nonexistent in fetuses or newborn infants. Transient abnormal myelopoiesis (TAM) is a benign fetal and neonatal form of myeloproliferative disorder. Another label for this condition is *acute leukemoid reaction*.[10] It, too, is often recognized in trisomy 21 and must be differentiated from congenital leukemia. In vitro assays for granulocyte macrophage colony-forming units (CFU-GM) are normal in TAM, whereas with leukemia, abnormal maturation is found.[11,12] In TAM, the peripheral blood may contain up to 90% blast forms. We had no peripheral blood in this stillborn fetus, but vessels in the tissues did not have blood with a significant increase in nucleated forms.

Myelodysplastic syndromes are extremely rare in infants, only two cases having been reported in patients less than 2 months old,[13] one of these in association with trisomy 21.[14] In another stillborn with trisomy 21, megakaryocytosis was found in the hepatic sinusoids.[15]

Neonatal or fetal infection is not always easily diagnosed. The usual inflammatory response, both clinically and morphologically, may be muted, especially in premature fetuses and infants. In a case such as this, a stillborn fetus, we had no peripheral blood to test for leukocytosis or a left shift in the differential count. Therefore, we depended on the demonstration of inflammatory foci in the tissues.

The placenta is usually available for evaluation in cases of fetal death. Evidence of chorioamnionitis is associated with true fetal infection in most cases. The many studies of these correlations leave one a bit bewildered. For example, Svensson et al found that when acute chorioamnionitis was demonstrated pathologically, only 50% of the fetuses and neonates were clinically infected and, conversely, only 28% of infected neonates had demonstrable acute chorioamnionitis and funisitis.[16] On the other hand, Romero et al reported that when chorioamnionitis was present, especially with funisitis and vasculitis, 86% of the amniotic fluids were infected and had positive culture results and, conversely 96% of culture-positive amniotic fluid samples had associated chorioamnionitis pathologically.[17] When a fetus or newborn baby is premature, ie, less than 34 weeks' gestation, infection is present in 85% of those with severe chorioamnionitis and umbilical vasculitis involving two or all three vessels.[18] The mechanism of death in fetuses is related, at least in part, to the reduced flow of blood through inflamed umbilical vessels.[19] Had we not had the placenta with the marked acute chorioamnionitis and funisitis, we would have been left with the marked granulopoiesis in the liver to establish the diagnosis. If we rule out leukemias, benign myeloproliferative syndromes, and myelodysplastic syndromes, all of which are exceedingly rare, we can be confident that infection was the cause of this fetus's problems. The hepatic subcapsular hematoma supports that conclusion. In our experience, these lesions are often associated with sepsis in the premature fetus or neonate.

DIAGNOSIS: Fetal infection with excessive granulopoiesis in the liver; a leukemoid reaction or transient abnormal myelopoiesis (TAM)

References

1. Singer DB. Hepatic erythropoiesis in infants of diabetic mothers: A morphometric study. *Pediatr Pathol* 1986;5:471–479.
2. Bhat AM, Scanlon JW. The pattern of eosinophilia in premature infants: A prospective study in premature infants using the absolute eosinophil count. *J Pediatr* 1981;98:612–616.
3. Rothberg AD, Cohn RJ, Argent AC, Sher R, Joffe M. Eosinophilia in premature neonates. *S Afr Med J* 1983;64:539–541.
4. Lewis DB, Wilson CB. Developmental immunology and role of host defenses in neonatal susceptibility to infection. In: Remington JS, Klein JO, eds. *Infectious Diseases of the Fetus & Newborn Infant*. 4th ed. Philadelphia: WB Saunders Co; 1995:20–98.
5. Stallmach T, Karolyi L. Augmentation of fetal granulopoiesis with chorioamnionitis during the second trimester of gestation. *Hum Pathol* 1994;25: 244–247.

6. Fong CT, Brodeur GM. Down's syndrome and leukemia: Epidemiology, genetics, cytogenetics, and mechanism of leukemogenesis. *Cancer Genet Cytogenet* 1987;28:55–76.
7. Gray ES, Balch NJ, Kohler H, Thompson WD, Simpson JG. Congenital leukaemia: An unusual cause of stillbirth. *Arch Dis Child* 1986;61:1001–1006.
8. Las Heras J, Leal G, Haust MD. Congenital leukemia with placental involvement: Report of a case with ultrastructural study. *Cancer* 1986;58:2278–2281.
9. Penchansky L, Krause JR. Myeloproliferative syndrome in childhood. *Pediatr Pathol* 1983;1:311–318.
10. Bain B. Down's syndrome: Transient abnormal myelopoiesis and acute leukaemia. *Leukemia Lymphoma* 1991;3:309–317.
11. Jiang C-J, Liang D-C, Tien H-F. Neonatal transient leukaemoid proliferation followed by acute myeloid leukaemia in a phenotypically normal child. *Br J Haematol* 1991;77:247–278.
12. Liang D-C, Ma S-W, Lu T-H, Lin S-T. Transient myeloproliferative disorder and acute myeloid leukemia: Study of six neonatal cases with long-term follow-up. *Leukemia* 1993;7:1521–1524.
13. McMullin MF, Chisholm T, Hows JM. Congenital myelodysplasia: A newly described disease entity. *Br J Haematol* 1991;79:340–342.
14. O'Donnell MR, Nademanee AP, Snyder DS, et al. Bone marrow transplantation for myelodysplastic and myeloproliferative disorders. *J Clin Oncol* 1987;5:1822–1826.
15. Gilson TP, Bendon RW. Megakaryocytosis of the liver in a trisomy 21 stillbirth. *Arch Pathol Lab Med* 1993;117:738–739.
16. Svensson L, Ingemarsson I, Mårdh P-A. Chorioamnionitis and the isolation of microorganisms from the placenta. *Obstet Gynecol* 1986;67:403–409.
17. Romero R, Salafia CM, Athanassiadis AP, et al. The relationship between acute inflammatory lesions of the preterm placenta and amniotic fluid microbiology. *Am J Obstet Gynecol* 1992;166:1382–1388.
18. Keenan WJ, Steichen JJ, Mahmood K, Altshuler G. Placental pathology compared with clinical outcome: A retrospective blind review. *Am J Dis Child* 1977;131:1224–1227.
19. Fleming AD, Salafia CM, Vintzileos AM, Rodis JF, Campbell WA, Bantham KF. The relationships among umbilical artery velocimetry, fetal biophysical profile, and placental inflammation in preterm premature rupture of the membranes. *Am J Obstet Gynecol* 1991;164:38–41.

Case Six

Contributed by Don B. Singer, MD
Providence, Rhode Island

History

This male was stillborn at 21 weeks' gestation and weighed 326 g. The placenta was pale and weighed 185 g. The mother's blood type was B, Rh positive. She had no untoward symptoms during this, her first pregnancy, but a gonococcus culture result was positive at the time of delivery. The mother was promptly and successfully treated for the gonococcal infection, which had no bearing on the death of the fetus.

Dr Singer: The liver is autolyzed. Ghost remnants of hepatocytes are less conspicuous than the abundant hematopoietic cells. Erythroid precursors predominate in the sinusoids (Figure 6–1). The nuclei of the erythroids have inclusions with peripheral condensation of the chromatin at the nuclear membrane (Figures 6–2 and 6–3). The inclusions are lavender or pale purple in the routine preparations stained with hematoxylin and eosin. Most of the nucleated erythroids contain inclusions. These are virtually diagnostic of human parvovirus B19 inclusions. Special in situ hybridization stains with digoxigenin-tagged parvovirus B19 primers confirmed the diagnosis.

In this case, excessive numbers of nucleated red blood cells circulated in the blood vessels of the fetus and the placenta. In hematoxylin-eosin–stained preparations, for reasons that are unclear, erythroid viral inclusions in the placenta are not as readily identified as are similar cells in the fetal tissues. The lung is usually more adequately preserved than most other organs in cases of macerated stillborn fetuses and is therefore preferred in a search for inclusion-bearing nucleated erythroids. In this case, numerous such cells were identified in the lung, adrenal gland, thymus, spleen, heart, and bone marrow.

Parvovirus is a single-stranded DNA virus, which in humans is cytopathic for nucleated red blood cell precursors. It is more commonly known as the causative agent for erythema infectiosum (fifth disease) in young children. It can also cause fleeting reticular rashes and mild arthritis in adults. Because the nucleated erythroblast is the primary target for this agent, parvovirus B19 is a dangerous pathogen in patients of any age with chronic anemia.[1–3] It causes an aplastic crisis when it attacks and destroys the erythropoietic cells, which are constantly proliferating in these patients. In immunocompromised patients, transient neutropenia[4] and chronic anemia[5] have been attributed to parvovirus B19 infection. Resistance to infection has been demonstrated in those rare individuals (1 in 200,000) who do not have P antigen on their erythroids. The P antigen is the cellular receptor for parvovirus B19, and while the receptor is present on many cell types, the virus replicates only in erythroid precursors that have P antigen.[6]

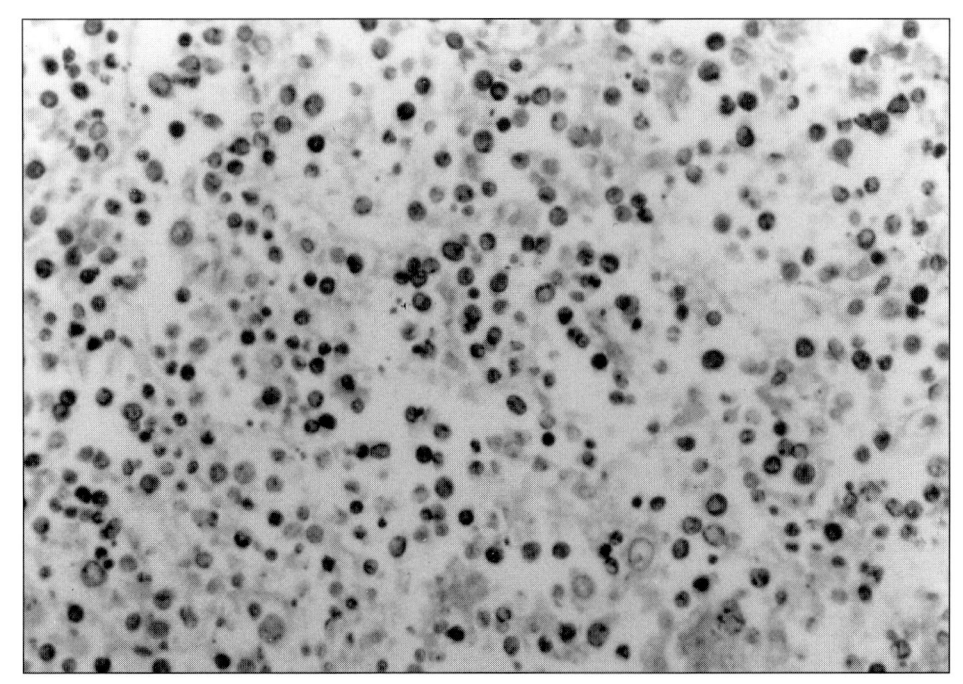

Figure 6–1. The autolyzed liver has innumerable erythroid precursors that are moderately well preserved. Pale remnants of hepatocytes are identified in the background.

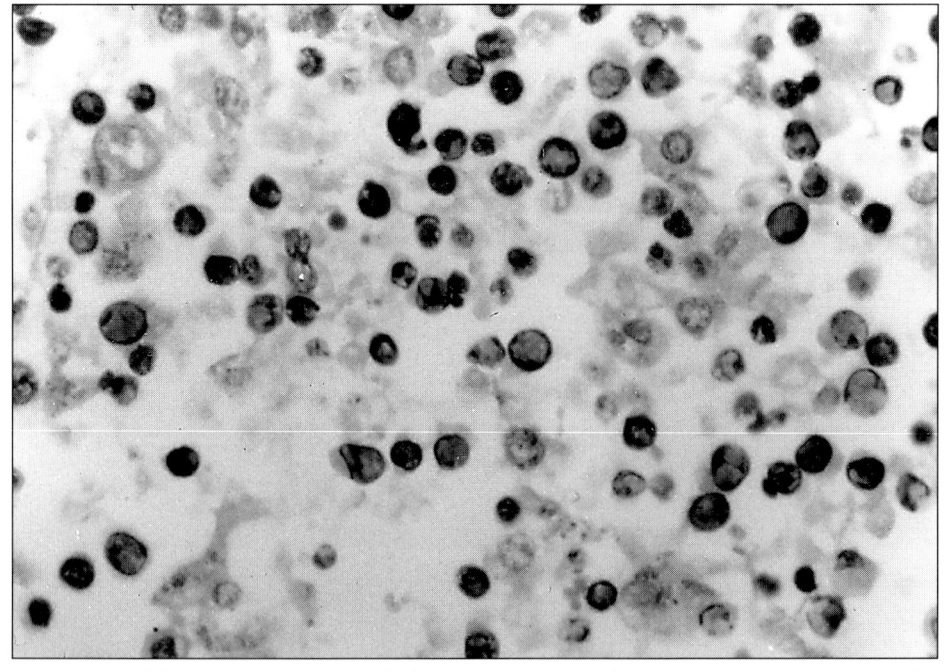

Figure 6–2. Nucleated erythroid cells have lightly stained intranuclear parvovirus inclusions and condensed chromatin at the edges of the nuclear membranes.

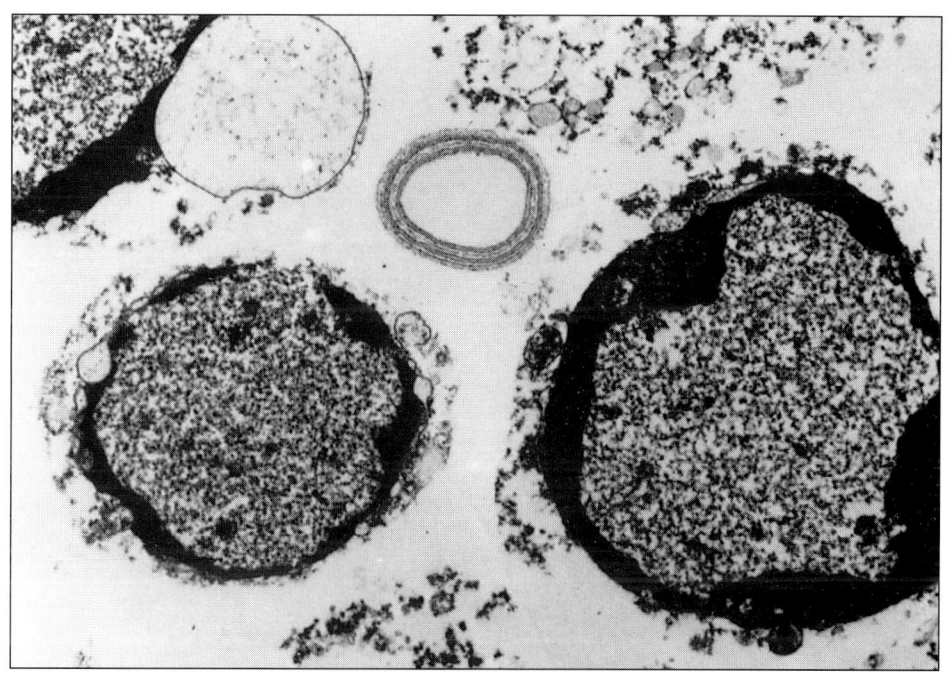

Figure 6–3. Electron micrograph with two nucleated erythroid cells and parvovirus inclusions. The edge of a larger third infected erythroid cell is present in the left upper corner of the photograph.

Although the evidence is tenuous, human parvovirus infections may have other target cells and tissues. Vasculitis has been reported in the placental villi.[7] In older children, necrotizing vasculitis has been associated with presumably chronic parvovirus B19 infection, but the virus may have been an opportunistic infection in these cases.[8] Active or recent parvovirus B19 infections were recently reported in children with Kawasaki disease.[9] Segmental proliferative glomerulonephritis has been reported in association with aplastic crisis and nephrotic syndrome in patients with sickle cell disease.[10] The cutaneous rash of fifth disease may represent a vasculitis, but this has yet to be shown histologically. In the many animal strains of parvovirus, which are distinct from the human B19 strain, the primary target cells and organs vary. The canine parvovirus targets myocardium, especially in puppies. Now and then, human B19 infections are reported with myocarditis and fatal damage to the heart,[11] but to date none of these cases has been proved with in situ hybridization of parvovirus B19 in myocardial cells. Such studies have shown conclusive proof for direct infection only in nucleated erythroids.[12,13]

Pallor and edema of the placenta and fetus suggest fetal anemia, but the differential diagnosis includes intrauterine infection. For example, syphilis will sometimes present with pallor and hydrops. Appropriate silver stains should be examined to establish the diagnosis in these cases. In decades past, Rh incompatibility between mother and fetus was the most common cause of these findings.

Bart's hemoglobinopathy (alpha-thalassemia with deletion of all four of the pertinent genes) must also be considered. Other mechanisms for these findings include intrauterine heart failure and blockade of lymphatic vessels, which sometimes occurs in Down syndrome. Others have reported chromosomal defects associated with parvovirus B19 and hydrops fetalis,[14] but these must be considered chance associations. Rogers et al examined autopsy materials retrospectively from 32 unselected cases of hydrops fetalis; 5 (15%) had parvovirus B19 infection as the cause. Only two of five placentas had diagnostic inclusions.[13] In this same series of cases, routine histologic studies with hematoxylin-eosin were as sensitive as molecular techniques in establishing the diagnosis. The molecular techniques, of course, add specificity not possible with routine histologic studies.[15]

In the 10 years or so since the first reported cases of fetal infection,[16] convincing evidence for a teratogenic role for parvovirus B19 has not been reported. Periodically, a case with malformations is found in the literature,[17] but the consensus is that the virus does not cause anomalies.[18-20] We prospectively examined 80 spontaneously aborted embryos and fetuses in the first trimester of gestation in an attempt to determine the incidence and possible causative role of parvovirus B19. Maternal serologic studies, routine histologic studies, electron microscopy, in situ hybridization, and polymerase chain reaction (PCR) techniques were used. Five mothers had seroconverted during pregnancy, and two of their abortuses had parvovirus B19 demonstrated in the aborted tissues with PCR studies. Only one of the two had intranuclear inclusions in erythroid precursors. In five specimens from mothers who did not have serologic evidence of infection (controls), false-positive inclusions were found in erythroid precursors in routine histologic preparations.[21] Since that study, we have seen isolated erythroids with presumed inclusions in abortuses but have not invoked a diagnosis of parvovirus infection unless the majority of nucleated erythroids are involved. Proof lies with maternal serologic studies or molecular diagnostic techniques.

Most cases of fetal parvovirus infection occur in early or midgestation when nucleated erythroid precursors are most numerous. A few cases have also been reported in the latter weeks of pregnancy. Infants may be liveborn[22] and some of these have residual lesions, such as marked siderosis in the liver, portal fibrosis, and proliferation of portal bile ducts.[23,24]

The prenatal diagnosis of intrauterine infection can be established in several ways. Maternal serologic studies have been used extensively with a rise in antiparvovirus B19 antibodies indicating an infection. Amniotic fluid can be tested with molecular probes specific for parvovirus B19.[25,26] Elevated maternal serum alpha-fetoprotein (AFP) may be the first evidence of disease, but by this time the fetus may be irreversibly damaged.[27] Krause et al have shown that if air-dried smears of peripheral blood are postfixed in formalin and stained with hematoxylin-eosin, the inclusions will be visible in nucleated red blood cells.[28]

More than half of the adult population in the United States have had parvovirus B19 infections and have IgG antibodies specific to that agent.[29] Approximately 1% of all pregnant women in the United States will have primary parvovirus B19 infection during gestation.[4] This figure may rise to as high as 6% during community epidemics.[19,30] Of those with primary infections, 33% will transmit the virus to their fetuses and an average of about 10% of these fetuses will have fatal disease. Another 25% will have symptoms of anemia. Immune globulins can be given to the mother[31] or directly to the fetus. Attempts to develop a vaccine have recently been reported.[32] Hall[33] has suggested the following clinical protocol to use in potential primary infections in pregnancy. The mother at risk should be tested serologically for parvovirus B19-specific IgM, IgG or DNA.[34] Retesting after 4 weeks is recommended. One impediment to such a program is the paucity of testing facilities.

Children and adults with typical rashes and arthralgias are no longer contagious, but HIV-positive patients or those with aplastic crisis may be regarded as infectious. In exposed fetuses with signs of anemia, intrauterine transfusions have been used with varying success.[19,35,36] The indications for treatment with intrauterine transfusions have not yet been defined.[33]

DIAGNOSIS: Fetal parvovirus B19 infection

References

1. Rao SP, Miller ST, Cohen BJ. Transient aplastic crisis in patients with sickle cell disease: B19 parvovirus studies during a 7-year period. *Am J Dis Child* 1992;146:1328–1330.
2. Mallouh AA, Qudah AK. Acute splenic sequestration together with aplastic crisis caused by human parvovirus B19 in patients with sickle cell disease. *J Pediatr* 1993;122:593–595.
3. Mallouh AA, Qudah AK. An epidemic of aplastic crisis caused by human parvovirus B19. *Pediatr Infect Dis J* 1995;14:31–34.
4. Koch WC, Adler SP. Human parvovirus B19 infections in women of childbearing age and within families. *Pediatr Infect Dis J* 1989;8:83–87.
5. Griffin TC, Squires JE, Timmons CF, Buchanan GR. Chronic human parvovirus B19-induced erythroid hypoplasia as the initial manifestation of human immunodeficiency virus infection. *J Pediatr* 1991;118:899–901.
6. Brown KE, Hibbs JR, Gallinella G, et al. Resistance to parvovirus B19 infection due to lack of virus receptor (erythrocyte P antigen). *N Engl J Med* 1994;330:1192–1196.
7. Morey AL, Keeling JW, Porter HJ, Fleming KA. Clinical and histopathological features of parvovirus B19 infection in the human fetus. *Br J Obstet Gynaecol* 1992;99:566–574.
8. Finkel TH, Török TJ, Ferguson PJ, et al. Chronic parvovirus B19 infection and systemic necrotising vasculitis: Opportunistic infection of aetiological agent? *Lancet* 1994;343:1255–1258.
9. Nigro G, Zerbini M, Krzystofiak A, et al. Active or recent parvovirus B19 infection in children with Kawasaki disease. *Lancet* 1994;343:1260–1261.
10. Wierenga KJJ, Pattison JR, Brink N, et al. Glomerulonephritis after human parvovirus infection in homozygous sickle-cell disease. *Lancet* 1995;346:475–476.
11. Porter HJ, Quantrill AM, Fleming KA. B19 parvovirus infection of myocardial cells. *Lancet* 1988;i:535–536.

12. Schwarz TF, Nerlich A, Hottenträger B, et al. Parvovirus B19 infection of the fetus: Histology and in-situ hybridization. *Am J Clin Pathol* 1991;96:121–126.
13. Rogers BB, Mark Y, Oyer CE. Diagnosis and incidence of fetal parvovirus infection in an autopsy series: I, Histology. *Pediatr Pathol* 1993;13:371–379.
14. Willekes C, Roumen FJME, Van Elsacker-Niele AMW, et al. Human parvovirus B19 infection and unbalanced translocation in a case of hydrops fetalis. *Prenatal Diagn* 1994;14:181–186.
15. Mark Y, Rogers BB, Oyer CE. Diagnosis and incidence of fetal parvovirus infection in an autopsy series: II, DNA amplification. *Pediatric Pathol* 1993;13:381–386.
16. Anand A, Gray ES, Brown T, Clewley JP, Cohen BJ. Human parvovirus infection in pregnancy and hydrops fetalis. *N Engl J Med* 1987;316:183–186.
17. Van Elsacker-Niele AMW, Vermeij-Keers C, Oepkes D, Van Roosmalen J, Gorsira MCB. A fetus with a parvovirus B19 infection and congenital anomalies. *Prenat Diagn* 1994;14:173–176.
18. Mortimer PP, Cohen BJ, Buckley MM. Human parvovirus and the fetus. *Lancet* 1985;2:1102.
19. Török TJ. Human parvovirus B19 infections in pregnancy. *Pediatr Infect Dis J* 1990;9:772–776.
20. Guidozzi F, Ballot D, Rothberg AD. Human B-19 parvovirus infection in an obstetric population. *J Reprod Med* 1994;39:36–38.
21. Rogers BB, Singer DB, Mak SK, Gary GW, Fikrig MK, McMillan PN. Detection of human parvovirus B19 in early spontaneous abortuses using serology, histology, electron microscopy, in situ hybridization, and the polymerase chain reaction. *Obstet Gynecol* 1993;81:402–408.
22. Berry PJ, Gray ES, Porter HJ, Burton PA. Parvovirus infection of the human fetus and newborn. *Semin Diagn Pathol* 1992;9:4–12.
23. Metzman R, Anand A, DeGiulio PA, Knisely AS. Hepatic disease associated with intrauterine parvovirus B19 infection in a newborn premature infant. *J Pediatr Gastroenterol Nutr* 1989;9:112–114.
24. White FV, Jordan J, Dickman PS, Knisely AS. Fetal parvovirus B19 infection and liver disease of antenatal onset in an infant with Ebstein's anomaly. *Pediatr Pathol Lab Med* 1995;15:121–129.
25. Rogers BB, Mak SK, Dailey JV, Saller DN Jr, Buffone GJ. Detection of parvovirus B19 DNA in amniotic fluid by PCR DNA amplification. *Biotechniques* 1993;15:406–408,410.
26. Török TJ, Wang Q-Y, Gary GW Jr, Yang C-F, Finch TM, Anderson LJ. Prenatal diagnosis of intrauterine infection with parvovirus B19 by the polymerase chain reaction technique. *Clin Infect Dis* 1992;14:149–155.
27. Saller DN, Rogers BB, Canick JA. Maternal serum biochemical markers in pregnancies with fetal parvovirus B19 infection. *Prenat Diagn* 1993;13:467–471.
28. Krause JR, Penchansky L, Knisely AS. Morphologic diagnosis of parvovirus B19 infection. *Arch Pathol Lab Med.* 1992;116:178–180.
29. Gillespie SM, Cartter ML, Asch S, et al. Occupational risk of human parvovirus B19 infection for school and day-care personnel during an outbreak of erythema infectiosum. *JAMA* 1990;263:2061–2065.

30. Rodis JF, Hovick TJ Jr, Quinn DL, Rosengren SS, Tattersall P. Human parvovirus infection in pregnancy. *Obstet Gynecol* 1988;72:733–738.
31. Selbing A, Josefsson A, Dahle LO, Lindgren R. Parvovirus B19 infection during pregnancy treated with high-dose intravenous gammaglobulin. *Lancet* 1995;345:660–661.
32. Anderson S, Momoeda M, Kawase M, Kajigaya S, Young NS. Peptides derived from the unique region of B19 parvovirus minor capsid protein elicit neutralizing antibodies in rabbits. *Virology* 1995;206:626–632.
33. Hall CJ. Parvovirus B19 infection in pregnancy. *Arch Dis Child* 1994;71:F4–5.
34. Soderlund M, Brown CS, Cohen BJ, Wedman K. Accurate serodiagnosis of B19 parvovirus infections by measurement of IgG avidity. *J Infect Dis* 1995;171:710–713.
35. Panero C, Azzi A, Carbone C, Pezzati M, Mainardi G, di Lollo S. Fetoneonatal hydrops from human parvovirus B19: Case report. *J Perinatal Med* 1994;22:257–264.
36. Schwarz TF, Roggendorf M, Hottenträger B, et al. Human parvovirus B19 infection in pregnancy. *Lancet* 1988;ii:566–567.

Case Seven

Contributed by Louis P. Dehner, MD
St Louis, Missouri

History

The patient was a 9-month-old male infant with failure to thrive, severe episodic vomiting, and developmental delay. He was the product of a pregnancy complicated by first trimester bleeding and gestational diabetes and was born to a 36-year-old G2 mother who had laryngeal polyps and required continuous positive airway pressure at night in the latter part of the pregnancy. At birth, the baby weighed 8 lb 3 oz and the Apgar scores were 7 and 9 at 1 and 5 minutes, respectively. When this baby was first seen clinically at 4 months of age, his weight was less than the birth weight. His 9 months of life were characterized by profound hypotonia, persistent feeding difficulties, and poor physical and mental development. Mild hepatomegaly was noted early in the clinical course and initial laboratory studies included bilirubin level, which was normal, and SGOT 375, SGPT 245, and LDH 444, all of which were abnormal. The creatine kinase level was normal. Liver and muscle biopsies were performed. At 8 months of age, he had his first seizure episode. Ascites developed, and over the course of the next 4 weeks, vomiting continued and the abdominal girth increased. Seizure activity increased and he died at 9 months of age.

Dr Dehner: The section of liver reflects the overall status of the liver at autopsy. The liver was shrunken, firm, and fibrotic and weighed 150 g (normal, 290 g). It had a pale yellow and micronodular appearance on cut section (Figure 7–1). Other gross findings included ascites, *Streptococcus pneumoniae* peritonitis, and a small brain weighing 650 g (normal, 820 g). The baby was severely cachectic, reflecting the fact that failure to thrive persisted throughout the patient's short existence.

Microscopically, there was a micronodular cirrhosis with panlobular fatty change and cholestasis (Figure 7–2). Bile duct proliferation was noted focally in the fibrotic septal areas. A liver biopsy specimen obtained approximately 2 months before death also showed diffuse microvesicular and macrovesicular steatosis and mild bridging fibrosis without evidence of cirrhosis (Figure 7–3). There was a mild chronic inflammatory infiltrate in some of the portal tracts. Focal hepatocellular necrosis was also present. The diagnostic impression of the liver biopsy specimen was that it was consistent with a metabolic hepatopathy, but its appearance did not suggest a specific inborn error of metabolism.

This infant even in death has remained a diagnostic enigma. In addition to failure to thrive, this baby manifested severe developmental delay, had persistent metabolic acidosis with mildly elevated serum levels of pyruvate and lactate,

Case Seven 39

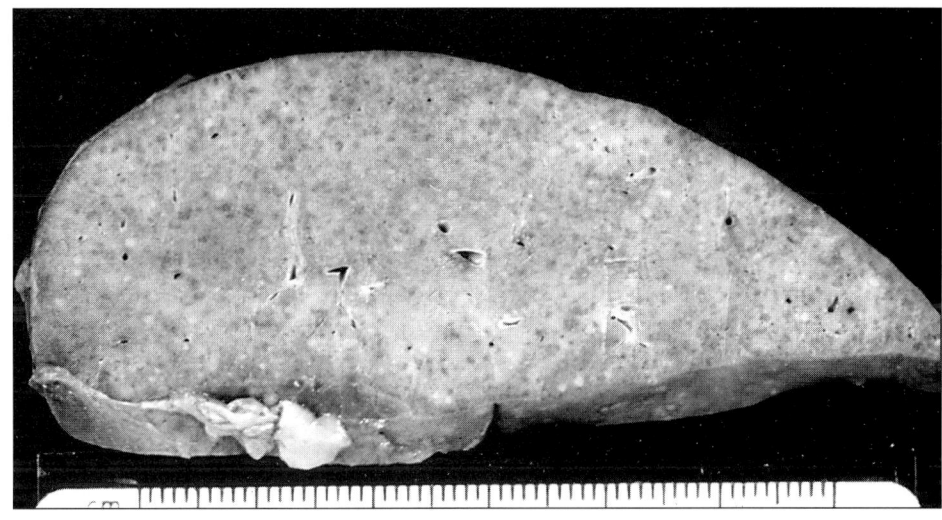

Figure 7–1. A pale yellow, finely nodular surface of the liver is shown in this cross section.

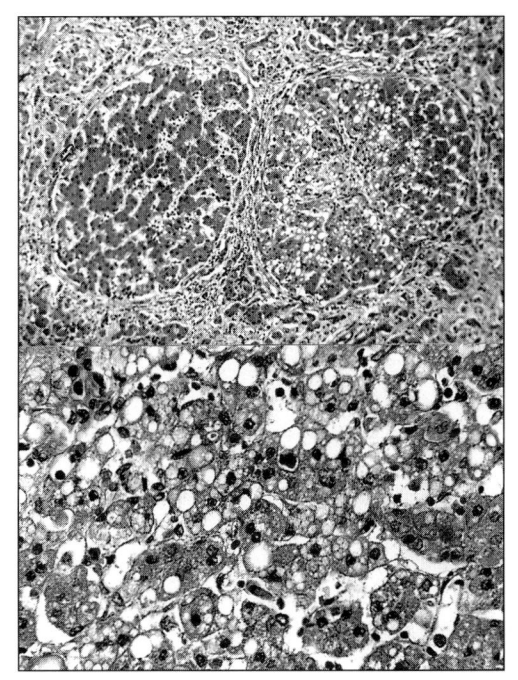

Figure 7–2. Uniformly small regenerative nodules are surrounded by fibrous bands containing numerous bile ducts (top). In addition to the fatty change, pseudoacinar transformation and cholestasis are findings not apparent in the previous liver biopsy specimen (bottom).

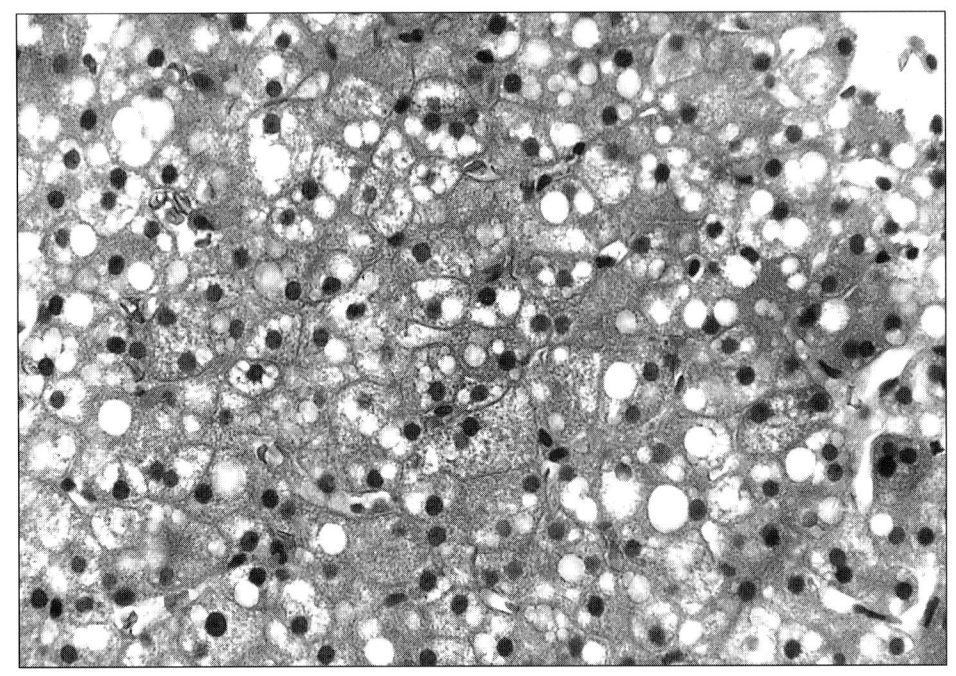

Figure 7–3. Liver biopsy specimen obtained 2 months before death shows predominantly microvesicular steatosis.

became jaundiced, and 2 months before death had the onset of seizures. Amino acid screening and determinations of peroxisomal and biotinidase activities failed to disclose any abnormalities. The carnitine level was mildly elevated, but the acylcarnitine profile was normal. Skin and muscle biopsy results failed to disclose any specific changes except for the fact that the type II muscle fibers were small.

Some complications occurred during the pregnancy, but the delivery was entirely unremarkable. This infant was seemingly normal in the initial weeks of life, but feeding difficulties developed and there was failure to gain weight. A clinical situation known as *failure to thrive* or *growth failure in infancy* had emerged to the extent that the weight at 4 months was less than the weight at birth. In addition to a weight below the third percentile, the height and head circumference were similarly affected.

Poor growth in infancy is relatively common in the underdeveloped areas of the world. In the United States and other western countries, a diagnostic evaluation to determine the underlying cause of failure to thrive in neonates is responsible for 1% to 5% of all children's hospital admissions.[1,2] A specific organic cause for the poor growth is identified in only 30% to 40% of infants. Urinary tract infection, various gastrointestinal anomalies, gastroesophageal reflux, and metabolic disorders or inborn errors of metabolism are some of the factors responsible for poor growth. More often, social and/or environmental difficulties are identified as major contributing factors to the failure of the infant's growth. Needless to say, there is considerable expenditure of resources in the laboratory evaluation of these infants.

Table 7–1. Hepatopathy Associated With Metabolic Disorders

Glycogen storage diseases: types Ia, Ib, II, III, IV, VI, IXa, IXb, IXe

Mucopolysaccharidoses

Defect in glycosaminoglycans
  Mucolipodoses
  Manosidosis
  Aspartylglucosaminuria

Defective endoplasmic storage
  Alpha-1-antitrypsin deficiency

Amino acidopathies
  Tryosinemia

Lipoprotein and lipid metabolism

Peroxisomal disorders

Mitochondrial cytopathies
  Alpers disease

Metal metabolism
  Wilson's disease
  Indian childhood cirrhosis
  Neonatal iron storage disease

Others
  Cystic fibrosis

As this baby's clinical course evolved, a number of metabolic disorders were considered in the differential diagnosis given the apparent hepatic involvement (Table 7–1). With the development of repeated vomiting, severe hypotonia, and seizures, the question of Alpers disease or progressive neuronal degeneration of childhood with hepatic failure was considered since several of the cardinal manifestations of this disorder were present in this infant (Table 7–2).[3-5] However, as the designation of this disorder implies, the principal pathosis of the brain involves the loss of neurons and spongiform changes in the cerebral cortex, brain stem, and cerebellum.[6] The white matter in Alpers disease is usually spared and the examination of the brain in our case revealed a more or less normal cerebral cortex, but there was severe bilateral mesial temporal sclerosis and the hippocampi and dentate gyri were virtually devoid of neurons. In these latter areas, there was marked gliosis associated with loss of neurons. The neuronal loss and gliosis extended beyond the hippocampus to the parahippocampal temporal cortex where there was also neuronal loss, gliosis, and collapse of the neuropil. Other areas of the cerebral cortex were intact. A second major finding in the brain was diffuse reactive gliosis of the telencephalic white matter indicative of a leukodystrophy; these findings were similar to perinatal telencephalic leukoencephalopathy, but there was no documentation of perinatal hypoxia in this infant.[7]

Table 7–2. Clinical Features of Alpers Disease*

Normal birth and neonatal period
Insidious onset of developmental delay and failure to thrive
Bouts of vomiting
Onset of seizures
Signs of overt liver disease variable
Low-density regions in occipital and posterior temporal lobes on CT
  with progressive gray and white matter atrophy
Death by 3 years of age
A mitochondrial cytopathy†

*Adapted from Harding et al.[3]
†The pathogenesis of Alpers disease as a disorder of mitochondria has not been established.

There is an extensive list of inborn errors of metabolism whose major clinical manifestations are hepatic and neurologic in nature. Most of the storage disorders have a dominant neurologic component with or without organomegaly. When there is hepatic involvement in Gaucher disease or Niemann-Pick disease, types B and C, it is generally restricted to infiltration or accumulation of storage material in the Kupffer cells without producing appreciable hepatic dysfunction except in Niemann-Pick disease, type C.[8,9] Likewise, in the mucopolysaccharidoses, mucopolysaccharides accumulate in the hepatocytes leading to hepatomegaly, but without functional impairment.

In contrast to most of the storage disorders, there are inborn errors with substantial neurologic and hepatic comorbidity.[9] A generally well-known condition in this category is Wilson's disease with coinvolvement of the liver and the central nervous system. It is difficult to be certain whether some of the urea cycle disorders with neurologic manifestations may not be the result of hyperammonemia secondary to hepatic dysfunction.

Cirrhosis in children has some of the same causes as cirrhosis in adults. Examples are posthepatitic B- and C-associated cirrhoses, which are important causes of chronic liver disease in some geographic areas without regard for age. On the other hand, the most common cause of cirrhosis in childhood in developed countries is extrahepatic biliary atresia (EHBA) with the secondary biliary cirrhosis. Approximately 50% of all liver transplantations in children are performed for EHBA-associated biliary cirrhosis.[10] Metabolic diseases or inborn errors of metabolism account for another 20% of liver transplantations in children. Alpha-1-antitrypsin deficiency is the most common metabolic disease in most series and represents 50% to 65% of all cases in this category. Tyrosinemia, Wilson's disease, and glycogen storage disease in aggregate account for most of the remaining cases requiring liver transplantation in children.[10] When there is substantial impairment of another organ system like the central nervous system in our patient, liver transplantation is not considered appropriate as a treatment option. An important exception to this statement about comorbidity is the child with cystic fibrosis who may be a reasonable candidate for lung and liver transplantations; this particular clinical situation is relatively uncommon since most children with cystic fibrosis do not have severe chronic liver disease.

Table 7–3. Metabolic Liver Disease Complicated by Cirrhosis

Alpers disease
Alpha-1-antitrypsin deficiency
Cystic fibrosis
Fructosemia
Galactosemia
Gaucher disease
Glycogen storage disease, types III and IV
Hemochromatosis (neonatal iron storage disease)
Wolman disease
Hepatic porphyria
Indian childhood cirrhosis
Niemann-Pick disease, type D
Trihydroxycoprostemic acid
Tyrosinemia
Wilson's disease

Most examples of cirrhosis in children have macronodular features, as illustrated by post-EHBA biliary cirrhosis, alpha-1-antitrypsin deficiency, Wilson's disease, glycogen storage disease, type IV or amylopectinosis, and fructosemia (Table 7–3). Indian childhood cirrhosis, galactosemia, tyrosinemia (early cirrhotic stage), neonatal iron storage disease, and Alpers disease are all accompanied by micronodular cirrhosis.[11] With the exception of Alpers disease, all of these disorders were systematically excluded in our patient with rather exhaustive laboratory testing.[12,13] As already noted, the changes in the brain were not typical of Alpers disease. However, there are some Alpers-like syndromes including hypoxic-epileptic conditions, hepatotoxicity secondary to valproic acid, and cases such as this with atypical pathologic findings at autopsy.[3]

Alpers disease is considered by some as one of a group of disorders with a defect in the mitochondrial respiratory chain.[11,12] Lactic acidosis is one of the biochemical hallmarks of these conditions. Most of these children are dead by 4 to 5 years of age. The defect probably exists in complex I of the electron transport protein complex in the mitochondriopathies or mitochondrial encephalomyopathies.[14] Since mitochondrial DNA is inherited through the ovum, Alpers disease and the other mitochondriopathies or cytopathies are inherited through the mother.[15,16]

The histologic combination of steatosis and cholestasis is a nonspecific and common finding in a liver biopsy specimen from an infant with metabolic liver disease; however, only a few of these conditions actually progress to cirrhosis. Metabolic hepatopathies whose natural history is progression to cirrhosis include tyrosinemia, type IV glycogen storage disease, alpha-1-antitrypsin deficiency, Wilson's disease, bile acid synthesis defects, Byler disease, cystic fibrosis, Alagille syndrome, and Alpers disease. This child may have had a mitochondrial cytopathy, but one that is not yet characterized.[17]

DIAGNOSIS: Alpers-like syndrome with micronodular cirrhosis and leukoencephalopathy

References

1. Berwick DM, Levy JC, Kleinerman R. Failure to thrive: Diagnostic yield of hospitalization. *Arch Dis Child* 1982;57:347-351.
2. Homer C, Ludwig S. Categorization of etiology of failure to thrive. *Am J Dis Child* 1981;135:848-851.
3. Harding BN, Alsanjari N, Smith SJM, et al. Progressive neuronal degeneration of childhood with liver disease (Alpers disease) presenting in young adults. *J Neurol Neurosurg Psychiatry* 1995;58:320-325.
4. Frydman M, Jager-Roman E, deVries L, et al. Alpers progressive infantile neuronal poliodystrophy: An acute neonatal form with findings of the fetal akinesia syndrome. *Am J Med Genet* 1993;47:31-36.
5. Harding BN. Progressive neuronal degeneration of childhood with liver disease (Alpers-Huttenlocher syndrome): A personal review. *J Child Neurol* 1990;5:273-287.
6. Sparaco M, Bonilla E, Mauro S, et al. Neuropathology of mitochondrial encephalomyopathies due to mitochondrial DNA defects. *J Neuropathol Exp Neurol* 1993;52:1-10.
7. Armstrong DD. Neonatal encephalopathies. In: Duckett S, ed. *Pediatric Neuropathology*. Baltimore: Williams and Wilkins; 1995:334-351.
8. Ishak KG. Pathology of inherited metabolic disorders. In: Balistrei WF, Stocker JT, eds. *Pediatric Hepatology*. New York: Hemisphere Publishing Corp; 1990:77-158.
9. Ishak KG, Sharp HL. Metabolic errors and liver disease. In: MacSween RNM, Anthony PP, Scheuer PJ, eds. *Pathology of the Liver*. 3rd ed. Edinburgh: Churchill Livingstone; 1994:123-218.
10. Ryckman FC, Ziegler MM, Pedersen SH, et al. Liver transplantation in children. In: Suchy FJ, ed. *Liver Disease in Children*. St Louis: Mosby; 1994: 930–950.
11. Narkewicz MR, Sokol RJ, Beckwith B, et al. Liver involvement in Alpers disease. *J Pediatr* 1991;119:260-267.
12. Rinaldo P. Laboratory diagnosis of inborn errors of metabolism. In: Suchy FJ, ed. *Liver Disease in Children*. St Louis: Mosby; 1994:294-308.
13. Sharp HL. Approach to the child with metabolic liver disease. In: Suchy FJ, ed. *Liver Disease in Children*. St Louis: Mosby; 1994:672-685.
14. Johns DR. Mitochondrial DNA and disease. *N Engl J Med* 1995;333:638-644.
15. Tritschler H-J, Medori R. Mitochondrial DNA alterations as a source of human disorders. *Neurology* 1993;43:280-288.
16. DeVivo DC. The expanding clinical spectrum of mitochondrial diseases. *Brain Dev* 1993;15:1-22.
17. Sokol RJ, Narkewicz MR. Mitochondrial hepatopathies. In: Suchy FJ, ed. *Liver Disease in Children*. St Louis: Mosby; 1994:888-896.

Case Eight

Contributed by Martin H. Matthews, MD
Marquette, Michigan

History

An 11-year-old boy presented with abdominal pain and was thought to have appendicitis clinically, however, a cystic hemorrhagic mass in the liver was found at surgery. The tumor had partially ruptured and bled into the abdominal cavity. A right hepatic lobectomy was done. Following multidrug chemotherapy, the patient has done well after 1 year.

Dr Dehner: As noted from the history, this boy presented in a dramatic and emergent fashion with acute abdominal pain and was found to have a bulging mass in the right lobe of the liver that had already partially ruptured, with free blood in the abdominal cavity. Grossly, the tumor was solitary and occupied the right lobe. The lobe with the tumor weighed 265 g. A tear was noted in the capsule of the liver. Upon sectioning, a 7 × 7 × 6 cm hemorrhagic and necrotic mass with circumscribed borders was identified (Figure 8–1). The nonhemorrhagic portions of the tumor had a whitish mucoid appearance and were distinct from the surrounding normal-appearing hepatic parenchyma.

Microscopically, this undifferentiated or poorly differentiated neoplasm was characterized by its heterogeneous patterns and variable cellular morphologic characteristics, ranging from uniform elliptical to spindle-shaped cells with some nuclear atypia and occasional mitotic figures to areas with a trabecular appearance resembling hepatocellular carcinoma (Figure 8–2, top and bottom). Large, anaplastic cells, some associated with intracellular and extracellular hyaline bodies, were noted focally (Figure 8–3). Extensive areas of this neoplasm were obscured by the hemorrhage and necrosis. One of the important diagnostic features was the presence of atypical-appearing bile ducts at the periphery or interface of the liver with the growth of malignant cells in the surrounding stroma; this pattern is somewhat reminiscent of adenosarcoma of the uterus (Figure 8–4). With the exception of the nuclei of the undifferentiated anaplastic cells, elsewhere the tumor cells had round-to-ovoid nuclei with uniformly delicate chromatin resembling the nuclei of clear cell sarcoma of the kidney. The background of the tumor varied from a myxoid to hyalinized appearance, in densely cellular foci, a stroma was not appreciated (Figure 8–5).

Regardless of the histologic pattern in a given area of this neoplasm, the tumor cells were strongly reactive for vimentin (Figure 8–6, top). On the other hand, the bile ducts at the periphery of the mass were the only structures to express cytokeratin (Figure 8–6, bottom). There was focal immunoreactivity for muscle-specific actin, alpha-1-antitrypsin, and KP-1 (CD68), but an absence of immunopositivity for alpha-fetoprotein (Figure 8–7).

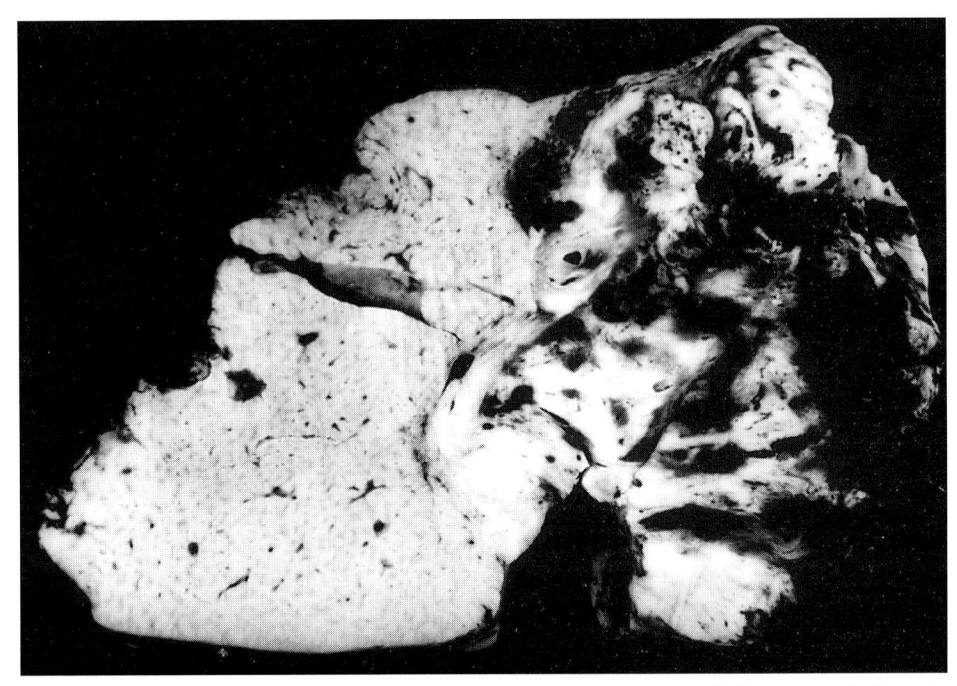

Figure 8–1. This partial hepatectomy specimen contains a well-demarcated, largely hemorrhagic mass. The gross appearance of this neoplasm readily explains the reason for its rupture before surgery.

As one compares the immunophenotype of the three neoplasms in the differential diagnosis of our case, hepatocellular carcinoma, rhabdomyosarcoma, and undifferentiated (embryonal) sarcoma (UES) (Table 8–1), it is readily apparent that hepatocellular carcinoma is no longer a sustainable diagnosis despite some histologic similarities. There was focal cellular immunopositivity for muscle-specific actin in our case, but other clinical, histologic, and immunohistochemical findings weighed unfavorably in terms of an embryonal rhabdomyosarcoma. Most rhabdomyosarcomas presenting in the region of the liver have originated

Table 8–1. Differential Immunohistochemistry of Hepatocellular Carcinoma, Rhabdomyosarcoma, and Undifferentiated (Embryonal) Sarcoma

Cancer Type	VIM	CK	EMA	MSA	DES	NSE	AAT	AFP
HCC	−	+	−	−	−	−	±	±
RMS	+	−	−	+	+	±	−	−
UES	±	±	−	±	±	±	±	−

Abbreviations: HCC = hepatocellular carcinoma; RMS = rhabdomyosarcoma; UES = undifferentiated (embryonal) sarcoma; VIM = vimentin; CK = cytokeratin; EMA = epithelial membrane antigen; MSA = muscle-specific actin; DES = desmin; NSE = neuron-specific enolase; AAT = alpha-1-antitrypsin; AFP = alpha-fetoprotein.

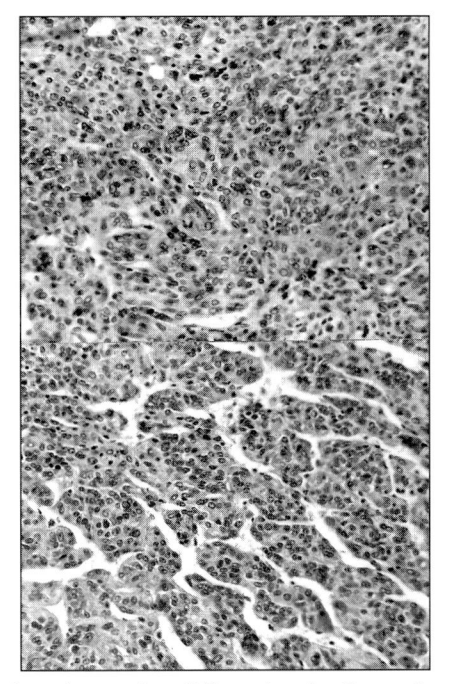

Figure 8–2. Solid, formless sheets of undifferentiated cells are the dominant histologic pattern (top), but other areas of the tumor strongly resemble hepatocellular carcinoma (bottom).

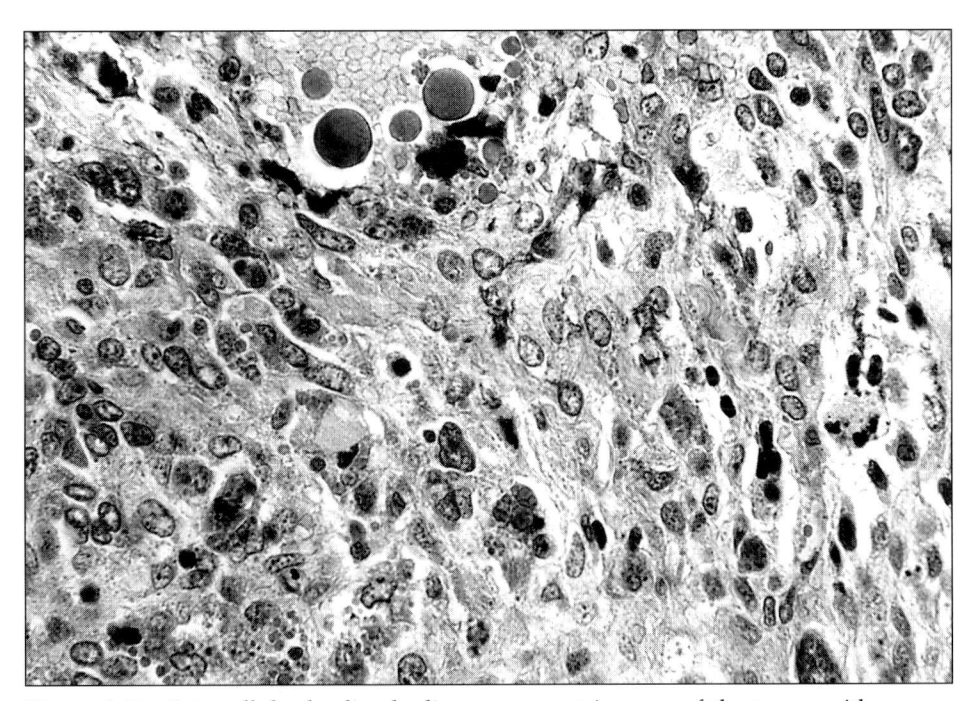

Figure 8–3. Extracellular hyaline bodies are present in areas of the tumor with a more pleomorphic population of malignant cells.

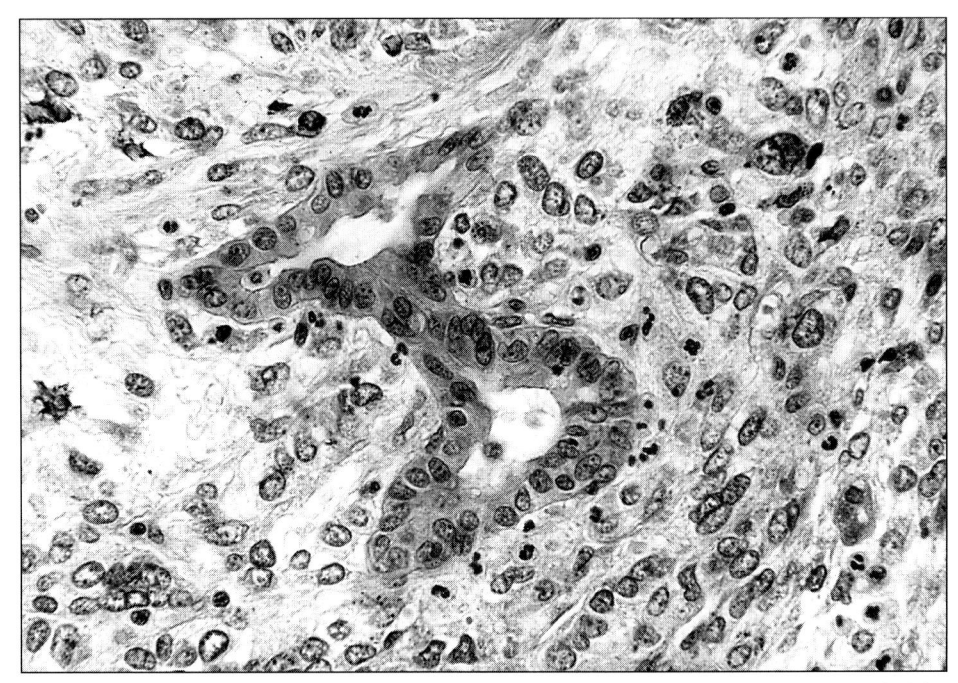

Figure 8–4. One of several bile ducts at the periphery of the tumor is surrounded by undifferentiated tumor cells in a myxoid or edematous background. The epithelium of the residual bile ducts may acquire reactive or atypical features, but the bile ducts are regarded as nonneoplastic in nature.

in the biliary tract of children between the ages of 1 and 5 years.[1] Obstructive jaundice and a mass in the porta hepatis are the other clinical features. If there is involvement of hepatic parenchyma, it is usually in the form of direct growth from the common bile duct or hepatic duct into the liver.

UES is a primary neoplasm of the liver with an overwhelming predilection for children, but with a few individual reports in adults.[2] This tumor was initially reported as a malignant mesenchymoma by Stanley et al[3] and later as a UES by Stocker and Ishak.[4] More than 50% of patients are between 6 and 10 years of age at presentation with acute abdominal pain and a mass.[5] The serum bilirubin level is generally not elevated, but some of the hepatic enzyme levels may be abnormal. A solitary, cystic, and/or hemorrhagic mass within the right lobe or a pedunculated mass is the usual gross appearance.[6,7] These tumors are typically quite large, generally in excess of 10 cm and 500 g. Microscopically, these tumors may show a range of features from loosely arranged, small, primitive spindle-to-stellate cells around small bile ducts at the periphery to solid sheets of cells, as demonstrated in our case. Immunohistochemistry has demonstrated the immunophenotypic heterogeneity of this neoplasm, including positivity for alpha-1-antitrypsin, vimentin, desmin, actin, cytokeratin, lysozyme, and neuron-specific enolase.[8–11] Alpha-1-antitrypsin and vimentin are expressed in 70% or more of cases whereas cytokeratin, desmin, and actin are detected in 25% to 30% of tumors. These tumors are typically nonreactive for epithelial

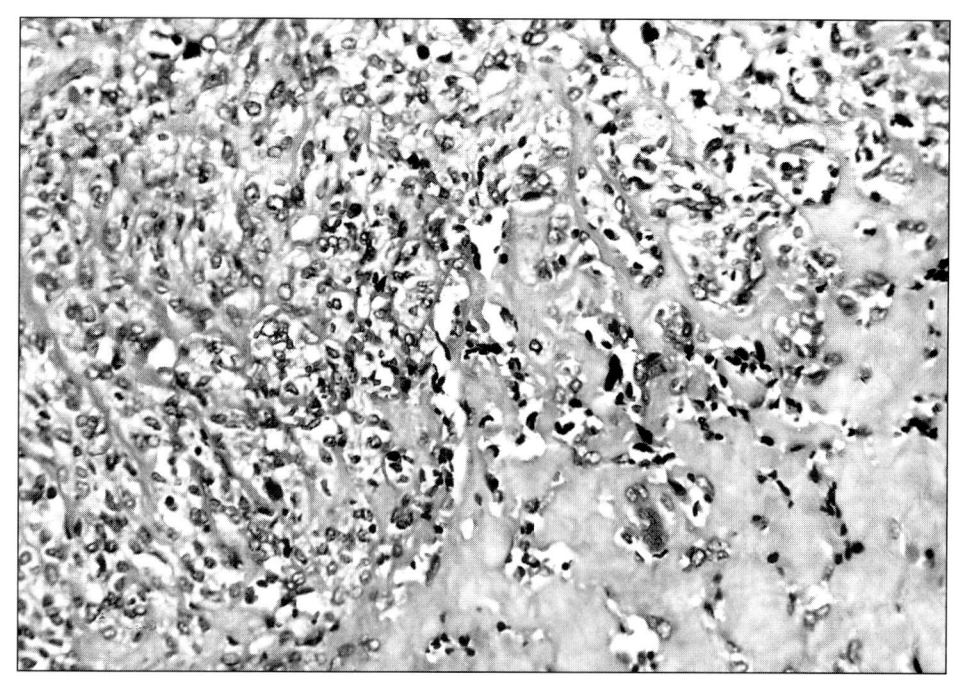

Figure 8–5. Other areas of the tumor have a hyalinized rather than a myxoid stroma or background. A similar hyalinized stroma may be seen in the hepatoblastoma, clear cell sarcoma of the kidney, and malignant renal rhabdoid tumor.

membrane antigen, alpha-fetoprotein, and carcinoembryonic antigen. Electron microscopy has not provided any insights into the differentiation or histogenesis of this tumor. Some have suggested that the UES is a fibrohistiocytic neoplasm.[12] We would conclude that this neoplasm is probably derived from uncommitted mesenchymal cells. There is an interesting case by deChadarevian et al, who reported the occurrence of a UES in conjunction with mesenchymal hamartoma of the liver.[13] There has been speculation in the past that the mesenchymal hamartoma is the progenitor of UES, but there have been few cases to support this hypothesis.[14]

Hepatoblastoma (27% of cases) and infantile hemangioendothelioma (19% of cases) are the two most common hepatic neoplasms in children to the age of 20 years (Table 8–2). UES accounted for only 7% of cases, but if one focuses on hepatic tumors presenting in the age range to which our patient belonged (5 to 20 years), then UES emerges as the second most common neoplasm to hepatocellular carcinoma (Table 8–3). Whereas the 2-year survival for hepatocellular sarcoma in children is 15% to 25%, the survival in the same period for UES has been less than 10%.[4,5] Failure of local control of tumor has been the principal cause of unfavorable outcome. However, few cases of long-term survival have been reported recently.[16–18] It is entirely possible that this boy will do well since most tumor relapses occur in the first year after diagnosis.

DIAGNOSIS: Undifferentiated (embryonal) sarcoma of the liver

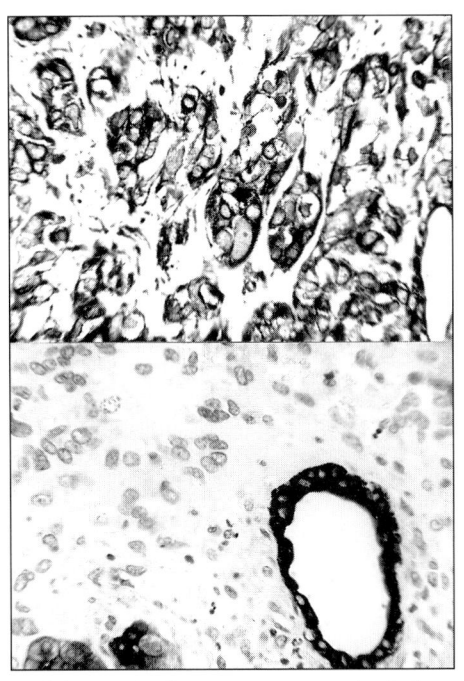

Figure 8–6. Regardless of the particular pattern or cytologic features, the tumor cells are universally immunoreactive for VIM (top), but only the peripheral bile ducts and entrapped hepatocytes show immunopositivity for cytokeratin (bottom).

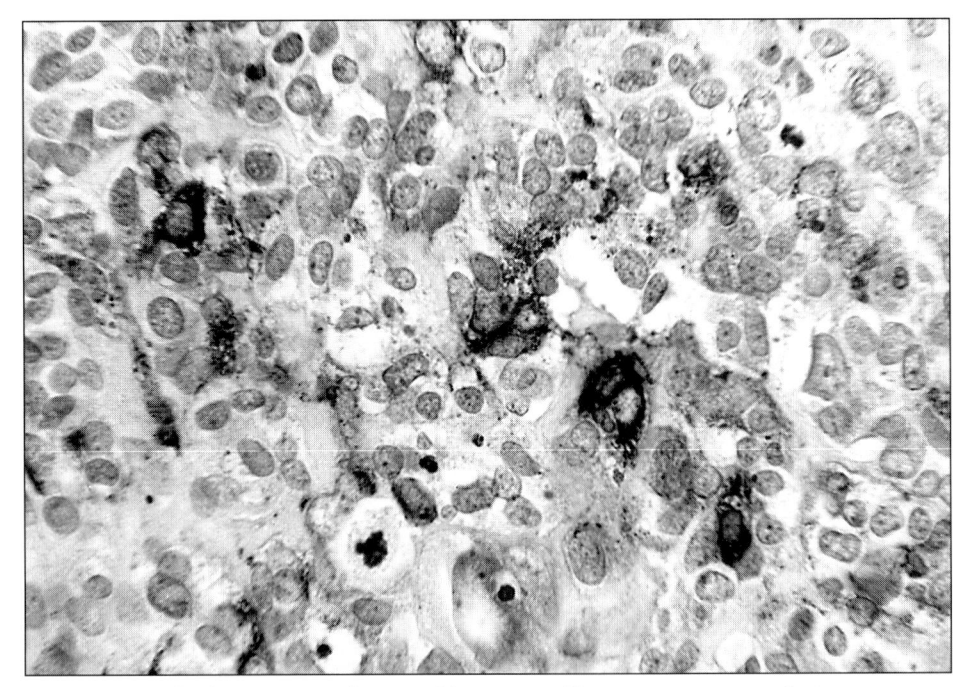

Figure 8–7. The larger, more pleomorphic tumor cells are more commonly immunoreactive for alpha-1-antitrypsin than are the smaller, undifferentiated cells.

Table 8–2. Types of Primary Hepatic Tumors Diagnosed in the First Two Decades of Life*

Type of Tumor	No.	%
Hepatoblastoma	167	26
Hepatocellular carcinoma	123	19
Infantile hemangioendothelioma	113	17
Focal nodular hyperplasia	63	10
Mesenchymal hamartoma	51	8
Undifferentiated "embryonal" sarcoma	46	7
Nodular regenerative hyperplasia	41	6
Hepatocellular adenoma	24	4
Angiosarcoma	13	2
Embryonal rhabdomyosarcoma	7	1
Total	648	~100

*Compiled by J Thomas Stocker, MD, 1995.

Table 8–3. Types of Primary Hepatic Tumors Diagnosed in Patients Between 5 and 20 Years of Age*

Type of Tumor	No.	%
Hepatocellular carcinoma	108	37
Focal nodular hyperplasia	52	18
Undifferentiated "embryonal" sarcoma	40	14
Nodular regenerative hyperplasia	32	11
Hepatocellular adenoma	23	8
Hepatoblastoma	17	6
Mesenchymal hamartoma	8	3
Angiosarcoma	5	2
Infantile hemangioendothelioma	4	1
Embryonal rhabdomyosarcoma	2	1
Total	291	~100

*Compiled by J Thomas Stocker, MD, 1995.

References

1. Roymahn FB, Rahey RB Jr, Crist WM, et al. Rhabdomyosarcoma of the biliary tree in childhood: A report from the Intergroup Rhabdomyosarcoma Study. *Cancer* 1985;56:575–581.
2. Johnson JA, White JG, Thompson AR. Undifferentiated (embryonal) sarcoma of the liver in adults. *Am Surg* 1995;61:285–297.
3. Stanley RJ, Dehner LP, Hesker AE. Primary malignant tumors (mesenchymoma) of the liver in childhood: An angiographic-pathologic study of three cases. *Cancer* 1973;32:973–984.

4. Stocker JT, Ishak KG. Undifferentiated (embryonal) sarcoma of the liver: Report of 3 cases. *Cancer* 1978;42:336–348.
5. Stocker JT. Hepatic tumors in children. In: Suchy FJ, ed. *Liver Disease in Children*. St Louis: Mosby; 1994:901–929.
6. Moon WK, Kim WS, Kim IO, et al. Undifferentiated embryonal sarcoma of the liver: US and CT findings. *Pediatr Radiol* 1994;24:500–503.
7. Ros PR, Olmstead WW, Dachman AH, et al. Undifferentiated (embryonal) sarcoma of the liver: Radiologic-pathologic correlation. *Radiology* 1986;161: 141–145.
8. Lack EE, Schloo BL, Azumi N, et al. Undifferentiated (embryonal) sarcoma of the liver: Clinical and pathologic study of 16 cases with emphasis on immunohistochemical features. *Am J Surg Pathol* 1991;15:1–16.
9. Aoyama C, Hachitanda Y, Sato JK, et al. Undifferentiated (embryonal) sarcoma of the liver: A tumor of uncertain histogenesis showing divergent differentiation. *Am J Surg Pathol* 1991;15:615–624.
10. Chou P, Mangkornkanok M, Gonzalez-Crussi F. Undifferentiated (embryonal) sarcoma of the liver: Ultrastructure, immunohistochemistry, and DNA ploidy analysis of two cases. *Pediatr Pathol* 1990;10:549–562.
11. Miettinen M, Kahlos T. Undifferentiated (embryonal) sarcoma of the liver: Epithelial features as shown by immunohistochemical analysis and electron microscopy. *Cancer* 1989;64:2096–2103.
12. Keating S, Taylor GP. Undifferentiated (embryonal) sarcoma of the liver: Ultrastructural and immunohistochemical similarities with malignant fibrous histiocytoma. *Cancer* 1985;16:693–699.
13. deChadarevian JP, Pawel BR, Faerber EN, Weintraub WH. Undifferentiated (embryonal) sarcoma arising in conjunction with mesenchymal hamartoma of the liver. *Mod Pathol* 1994;7:490–493.
14. Otal TM, Hendricks JB, Pharis P, Donnelly WH. Mesenchymal hamartoma of the liver: DNA flow cytometric analysis of eight cases. *Cancer* 1994;74: 1237–1242.
15. Perilongo G, Carli M, Sainati L, et al. Undifferentiated (embryonal) sarcoma of liver in childhood: Results of a retrospective Italian study. *Tumori* 1989; 73:213–217.
16. Urban LE, Mache W, Schwinger W, et al. Undifferentiated (embryonal) sarcoma of the liver in childhood: Successful combined-modality therapy in four patients. *Cancer* 1993;72:2511–2516.
17. Walker NI, Horn MJ, Strong RW, et al. Undifferentiated (embryonal) sarcoma of the liver: Pathologic findings and long-term survival after complete surgical resection. *Cancer* 1992;69:52–59.
18. Horowitz ME, Etcubanas E, Webber BL, et al. Hepatic undifferentiated (embryonal) sarcoma and rhabdomyosarcoma in children: Results of therapy. *Cancer* 1987;59:396–402.

Case Nine

Contributed by Robert W. Novak, MD
Akron, Ohio

History

This infant's mother had sudden abdominal pain, and he was delivered by cesarean section for possible placental abruption at 35 weeks' gestation. He was sent home, apparently normal, at 3 days of age but returned 2 days later with jaundice and pallor. His alanine aminotransferase (ALT) level was elevated and the total bilirubin level was 166 µmol/L. The platelet count was 24×10^9/L. Apneic episodes, seizures, and cardiac arrhythmias developed. Massive, fatal pulmonary hemorrhage developed at 8 days of age.

Dr Singer: The liver was not enlarged and macroscopically had no hint of necroses. Microscopically, diffusely scattered bland hepatic necroses have a minimal inflammatory cell response (Figure 9–1). The necrotic patches are unrelated to lobular architecture; they are neither centrolobular, midlobular, nor periportal. Portal tracts tend to be spared, but some are caught in the field of necrosis. Scattered through the viable parenchyma are occasional multinucleated cells. Extrahepatic lesions include pneumonitis and, coupled with the thrombocytopenia, this evolved into the fatal episode of pulmonary hemorrhage. The hemorrhage was both interstitial and intraalveolar. Lymphocytic meningitis was moderately severe (Figure 9–2). Focal necroses were identified in the heart (Figure 9–3), bone marrow, cerebrum, and pancreas. The placenta was unavailable for study.

The differential diagnosis in this case includes neonatal hepatitis, giant cell hepatitis (transformation), syphilis, cytomegalovirus infection, herpes simplex infection, enterovirus infection, and parvovirus B19 infection. With this clinical picture and histologic pattern of hepatic necrosis, the list of possibilities can be quickly narrowed to herpes simplex infection, echovirus infection, or coxsackievirus infection. All three of these infectious agents can produce meningitis and hepatitis with lesions in the other viscera as previously described. The clinical features in this baby included a brief interlude of apparently normal health followed by rapid deterioration and thrombocytopenia with fatal hemorrhage at 8 days of age. Herpes simplex, echoviruses, or coxsackieviruses can produce this characteristic clinical course.[1] The episode of maternal abdominal pain prior to the baby's birth may also have been an acute infectious illness, clinically most consistent with an enteroviral infection.[2]

Herpes simplex virus can infect the fetus in utero but more often is transmitted during parturition. This is compatible with the clinical story in this case, with or without evidence of maternal genital herpes infection. However, the herpes

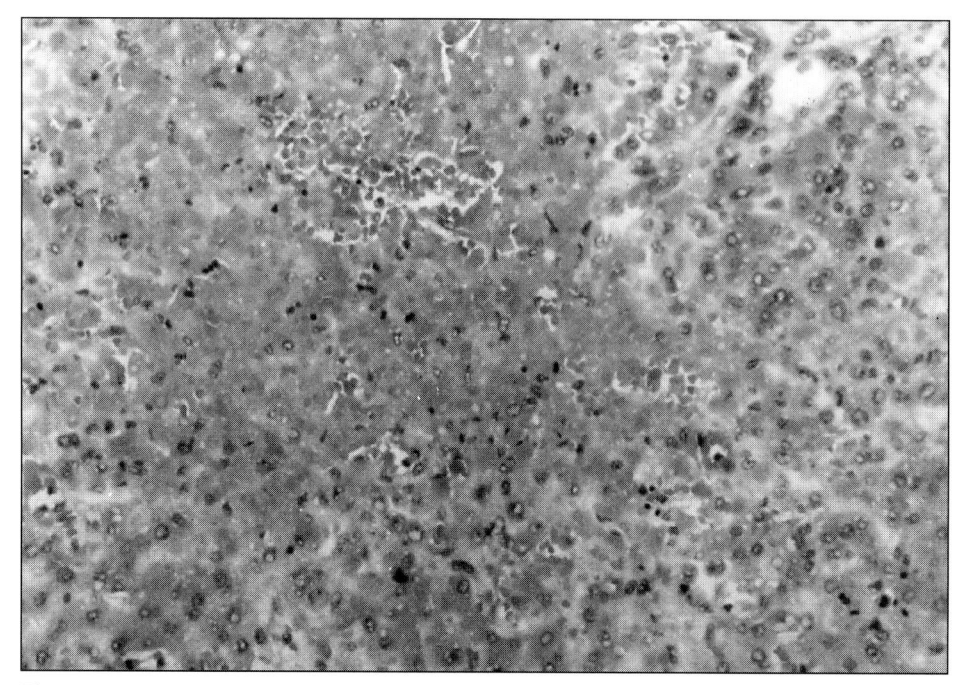

Figure 9–1. Hepatic necrosis is unattended by inflammatory reaction. The edges of the illustration show viable hepatocytes.

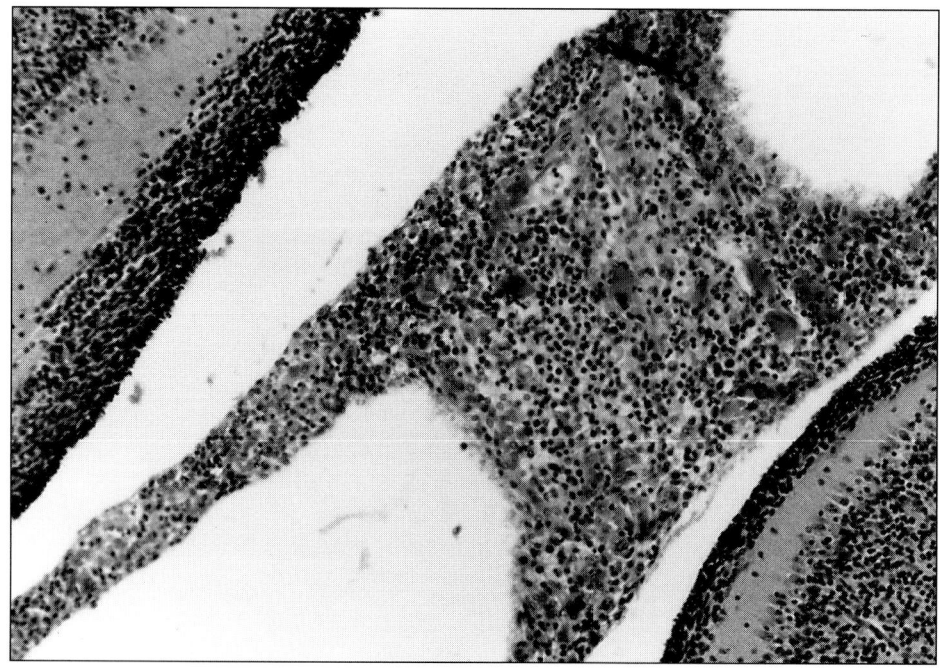

Figure 9–2. Lymphocytic meningitis in the cerebellar meninges. Foci of necrosis were present throughout the brain.

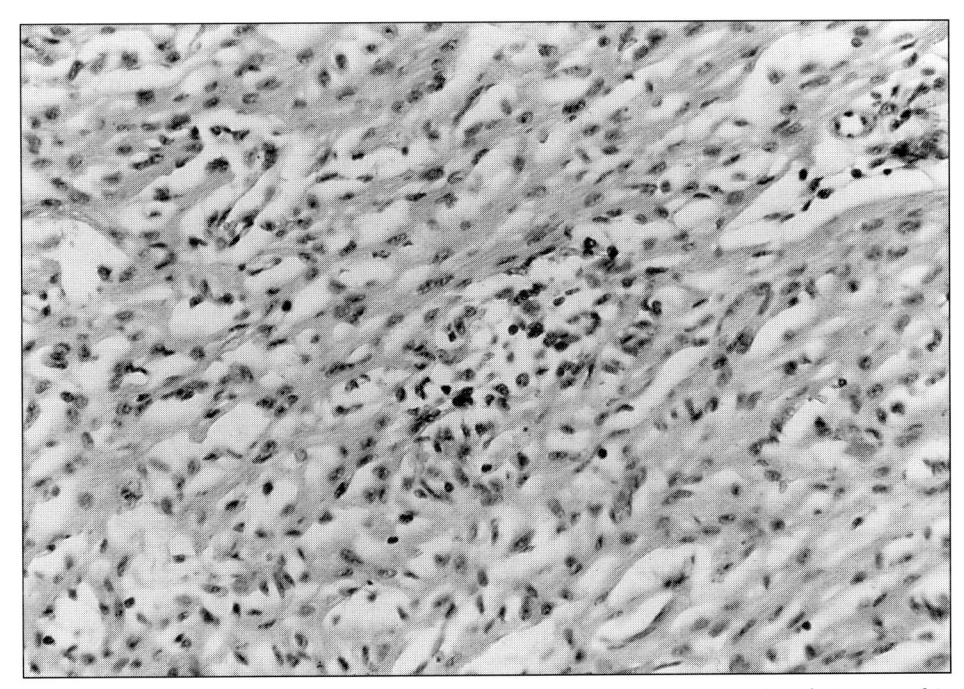

Figure 9–3. Myocardial necrosis and lymphocytic infiltration is another feature in this case of neonatal coxsackievirus B1 infection.

simplex viruses produce easily detected intranuclear inclusions in the tissues, including surviving hepatocytes, so this diagnosis can be discarded on histopathologic grounds.[3]

Enteroviral infections in late pregnancy are common, especially during community outbreaks. Such infections are usually not serious for mothers or their fetuses, but as many as 65% of mothers are symptomatic if their babies have positive culture results for enteroviruses. Intrauterine enteroviral infection develops rarely early in gestation.[4] Echoviruses and coxsackievirus B infections are not associated with spontaneous abortions, but stillbirths late in pregnancy are described.[5] Between 30% and 50% of infected mothers will transmit the enteroviruses through the placenta to their babies; ascending infection from the vagina to the amniotic sac probably does not occur. The frequency of intrauterine transmission is unknown but most neonatal infections are acquired during or after birth. Transmission is either from the mother or other caretakers, by human-to-human contact, especially those in the hospital nursery where other babies or personnel may be infected.[6,7] Severity of illness ranges from asymptomatic to fatal disease.[8] Neonates may have exanthems, enanthems, pneumonia, gastroenteritis, necrotizing enterocolitis, hepatitis, pancreatitis, myocarditis, meningoencephalitis, generalized hemorrhage, shock, and sudden death. Approximately 35% of neonatal coxsackievirus B infections occur in premature infants. Those with the most severe disease have onset before 10 days of age. The most seriously affected infants have involvement of the brain and the heart or both. The baby under discussion had an overwhelming hepatitis syndrome. This is usually seen with echoviruses, but it has been reported with coxsackievirus B1[9] and B3.[10]

Severity of disease depends on several factors including the virus strain, mode of transmission, and passive immunity from the mother's antibodies.[5] Intravenous immunoglobulin has been used therapeutically with success.[8,11]

Enteroviruses belong to the Picornaviridae and are single-stranded RNA structures. Enteroviruses have diameters ranging from 24 to 30 nm and consist of naked protein capsids around a small dense RNA core. All enteroviruses are protected from nucleases by these protein coats that determine, among other things, antigenicity. The enteroviruses include the polioviruses 1-3; coxsackievirus A, 1-24; coxsackievirus B, 1-6; and echoviruses 1-34.[6] Although virtually all major enterovirus types have been reported in fetuses and newborn infants,[5] in the clinical setting of this case, poliovirus and coxsackievirus A can be discarded as causative agents. Many of the multiple strains of coxsackievirus B and of the echoviruses can produce the signs and symptoms found in this baby.[9,10,12]

The exact diagnosis of viral species can be performed on viral isolates or, using molecular techniques, on tissue specimens. Bowles et al have established the diagnosis of coxsackievirus B from myocardial biopsy specimens.[13]. Redline et al successfully diagnosed enteroviral infections using paraffin-embedded liver and cardiac tissues and polymerase chain reaction techniques.[14] Gauntt et al used coxsackie viral-specific antibodies on cells from the ventricular fluid of the brain,[15] while Schlesinger et al used cerebrospinal fluid and polymerase chain reactions with appropriate molecular probes to establish the diagnosis in several cases of infantile enteroviral meningitis.[16]

The lesions identified in postmortem examinations from echoviruses include hepatic and adrenal necroses with little inflammatory reaction, as was seen in this case. Reports of fatal neonatal infections with echoviruses 6, 11, and 19 emerged in the early and mid-1970s[17-19] and continued into the subsequent decade.[20] Other echoviruses with similar findings in neonates are echovirus 7, 14, and 21.[21,22] Hepatic involvement was particularly pronounced in these cases. Up to 95% of the liver may be necrotic but the reticulum network and extramedullary hematopoietic tissue are preserved. Virions measuring 16 to 18 nm in diameter are sometimes arranged as crystalloids.[23] Hepatic giant cells are only occasionally seen in these infections.[24]

Necrotic and inflammatory lesions are also seen in several other organs, chiefly the brain. Encephalitis consists of glial reaction, necrotic neurons, and perivascular lymphocytic infiltrates.[17] The adrenal gland may have necrotic lesions without much inflammation.[21] Purpuric skin lesions, mucosal hemorrhages in the gastrointestinal tract, pleural and peritoneal serosal hemorrhages, and visceral hemorrhages in the renal medulla, adrenal gland, heart, brain, and meninges are all described with echovirus infections.[23,25]

Coxsackievirus B infections, more than echovirus infections, tend to involve the heart. The lesions are multiple myocardial necroses and lymphocytic infiltrates. The left ventricle is more often involved than the right ventricle and pericarditis is often an associated lesion.[21] In experiments with mice, Gauntt et al produced sustained myocarditis without sustained virus replication and they suggest that antibodies to portions of the viral capsid mediate the inflammation in the heart.[26]

The pancreas is often inflamed when infected with coxsackievirus B.[27] Islets of Langerhans and interstitial tissues may have intense mononuclear infiltrates,[28] leading to the speculation that these infectious agents are responsible for some cases of diabetes mellitus in infancy or childhood.[27,29,30]

In enteroviral infections, placental involvement is rarely seen. Extensive perivillous fibrin deposits and villous necrosis with inflammation were described by Baltcup et al in a rare case with intrauterine coxsackievirus A infection.[4] Garcia et al[31] found villous necrosis, chronic villitis, and intervillositis in coxsackievirus B infections, but Benirschke and Kaufman claim that no meaningful lesions associated with enterovirus infections occur in placentas.[32] In this case the placenta was not submitted for pathologic examination.

Hepatitis associated with hemorrhagic pneumonia and lymphadenitis is described in one case of coxsackie B infection.[33] While echoviruses involve the liver more than do coxsackieviruses, in this case the exception proved the rule, since the diagnosis was coxsackievirus B1.

DIAGNOSIS: Neonatal coxsackievirus B1 infection

References

1. Druyts-Voets E, Van Renterghem L, Gerniers S. Coxsackie B virus epidemiology and neonatal infection in Belgium. *J Infection* 1993;27:311-316.
2. Baker DA, Phillips CA. Maternal and neonatal infection with coxsackie virus. *Obstet Gynecol* 1980;55:12s-15s.
3. Singer DB. Pathology of neonatal herpes simplex virus infection. *Perspect Pediatr Pathol* 1981;6:243-278.
4. Baltcup G, Holt P, Hambling MH, Gerlis LM, Glass MR. Placental and fetal pathology in coxsackie virus A9 infection: A case report. *Histopathology* 1985;9:1227-1235.
5. Modlin JF. Perinatal echovirus and group B coxsackievirus infections. *Clin Perinatol* 1988;15:233-247.
6. Cherry JD. Enteroviruses. In: Remington JS, Klein JO, eds. *Infectious Diseases of the Fetus and Newborn Infant.* 4th ed. Philadelphia: WB Saunders Co; 1995:404-446.
7. Wright HT Jr, Okuyama K, McAllister RM. An infant fatality associated with coxsackie B1 virus. *J Pediatr* 1963;63:428.
8. Isacsohn M, Eidelman AI, Kaplan M, et al. Neonatal coxsackievirus group B infections: Experience of a single department of neonatology. *Israel J Med Sci* 1994;30:371-374.
9. Kaplan MH, Klein SW, McPhee J, Harper RG. Group B coxsackievirus infections in infants younger than three months of age: A serious childhood illness. *Rev Infect Dis* 1983;5:1019-1032.
10. Krajden S, Middleton PJ. Enterovirus infections in the neonate. *Clin Pediatr* 1983;22:87-92.
11. Valduss D, Murray DL, Karna P, Lapour K, Dyke J. Use of intravenous immunoglobulin in twin neonates with disseminated coxsackie B1 infection. *Clin Pediatr* 1993;32:561-563.

12. Haddad J, Gut JP, Wendling MJ, et al. Enterovirus infections in neonates: A retrospective study of 21 cases. *Eur J Med* 1993;2:209-214.
13. Bowles NE, Richardson PJ, Olsen EGJ, Archarel LC. Detection of coxsackie-B-virus-specific RNA sequences in myocardial biopsy samples from patients with myocarditis and dilated myocardiopathy. *Lancet* 1986;i:1120-1123.
14. Redline RW, Genest DR, Tycko B. Detection of enteroviral infection in paraffin-embedded tissue by the RNA polymerase chain reaction technique. *Am J Clin Pathol* 1991;96:568-571.
15. Gauntt CJ, Gudrangen RJ, Brans YW, Marlin AE. Coxsackievirus group B antibodies in the ventricular fluid of infants with severe anatomic defects in the central nervous system. *Pediatrics* 1985;76:64-68.
16. Schlesinger Y, Sawyer JH, Storch GA. Enteroviral meningitis in infancy: Potential role for polymerase chain reaction in patient management. *Pediatrics* 1994;94:157-162.
17. Philip AGS, Larson EJ. Overwhelming neonatal infection with echo 19 virus. *J Pediatr* 1973;82:391-397.
18. Krous HF, Dietzman D, Ray CG. Fatal infection with echovirus types 6 and 11 in early infancy. *Am J Dis Child* 1973;126:842-846.
19. Lake AM, Lauer BA, Clark JC, Wesenberg RL, McIntosh K. Enterovirus infections in neonates. *J Pediatr* 1976;89:787-791.
20. Berry PJ, Nagington J. Fatal infection with echovirus 11. *Arch Dis Child* 1982;57:22-29.
21. Singer DB. Infections of fetuses and neonates. In: Wigglesworth JS, Singer DB, eds. *Textbook of Fetal and Perinatal Pathology.* Boston: Blackwell Scientific Publishers, Inc; 1991:525-591.
22. Georgieff MK, Belani K, Johnson DE, Thompson TR, Ferreieri P. Fulminant hepatic necrosis in an infant with perinatally acquired echovirus 21 infection. *Pediatr Infect Dis* 1987;6:71-73.
23. Hughes JR, Wilfert CM, Moore M, Benirschke K, Hoyos-Guerara E. Echovirus 14 infection associated with fetal necrosis. *Am J Dis Child* 1972;123:61-67.
24. Dimmick JE. Liver disease in the perinatal infant. In: Wigglesworth JS, Singer DB, eds. *Textbook of Fetal and Perinatal Pathology.* Boston: Blackwell Scientific Publishers Inc; 1991:981.
25. Mostoufi-Zadeh M, Lack E, Gang DL, Perez-Atayde A, Driscoll SG. Postmortem manifestations of echovirus 11 sepsis in five newborn infants. *Hum Pathol* 1983;14:818-823.
26. Gauntt CJ, Arizpe HM, Higdon AL, et al. Molecular mimicry, anti-coxsackievirus B3 neutralizing monoclonal antibodies, and myocarditis. *J Immunol* 1995;154:2983-2995.
27. Rosenberg HS, Kohl S, Vogler C. Viral infections of the fetus and the neonate. In: Naeye RL, Kissane JM, Kaufman N, eds. *Perinatal Diseases.* Baltimore, Md: Williams & Wilkins; 1981:133-200(monograph no. 22).
28. Ahmad N, Abraham AA. Pancreatic isleitis with coxsackie virus B5 infection. *Hum Pathol* 1982;13:661-662.
29. Jenson AB, Rosenberg HS, Notkins AL. Pancreatic islet-cell damage in children with fatal viral infections. *Lancet* 1980;ii:354-358.
30. Bolande RP. The pathology and pathogenesis of juvenile diabetes mellitus. *Perspect Pediatr Pathol* 1979;5:269-291.

31. Garcia AG, Basso NG, Fonseca MEF, Outanni HN. Congenital echovirus infection: Morphological and virological study of fetal and placental tissue. *J Pathol* 1990;160:123-127.
32. Benirschke K, Kaufmann P. *Pathology of the Human Placenta.* 2nd ed. New York: Springer-Verlag; 1990:595-596.
33. Castleman B, McNeely BU. Case records of the Massachusetts General Hospital: Case #20-1965. *N Engl J Med* 1965;272:907-914.

Case Ten

Contributed by Don B. Singer, MD
Providence, Rhode Island

History

This 18-month-old girl had swallowing difficulties and on radiograph had a large multicystic lesion of the right lung.

Dr Singer: The patient had thoracic surgery to close an aortic-pulmonary window at 1 month of age. When she was 9 months of age, a small cyst in the right posterior hemithorax, similar to the lesion under discussion, was removed. Because of the difficult surgical approach from the left (she had a right aortic arch), the lesion was incompletely excised. It recurred and grew to 15 cm in diameter before it was completely removed. The sections are of the recurrent cyst.

The wall of the cyst is largely collagenous but in some sections, smooth muscle layers have interposed clusters of ganglion cells. The cyst's lining varies from cuboidal cells in some sections to columnar cells in others. Ciliated pseudostratified columnar epithelium is present in some of the slides (Figure 10–1). Pancreas with both exocrine and endocrine components is found in many of the sections (Figure 10–2). Microscopic cysts are lined by varying gastrointestinal epithelial cells, predominantly with gastric differentiation (Figure 10–3). Chronic inflammation and fibrosis involve large portions of the cyst's wall. In some sections, tags of normal lung tissue are present. Hepatic tissue is not identified.

Clinically and radiographically, the cyst seemed to be in the lung. The differential diagnosis in this case included congenital cystic adenomatoid malformation of the lung (CCAM), hyperlucent lung, congenital lobar emphysema, sequestration of the lung, and foregut cyst. The last term is closely related to thoracic enteric (esophageal) duplication cysts and neurenteric cysts. (The terms *cysts* and *duplications* have been used more or less interchangeably, although some authorities would make a distinction based on lack of full differentiation in foregut cysts vs differentiated epithelium, eg, gastric, esophageal, or ciliated in duplications.[1]) Less likely clinical or radiologic diagnoses include mediastinal lesions such as cystic tumors of the thymus or neural tissues (eg, ganglioneuroma, neuroblastoma), pericardial cyst, or a teratoma. Most of these lesions would not be located laterally in the chest as was this lesion.[2] At surgery, the wall of the cyst was adherent to lung tissue but the lung was not invaded nor was it thought to be the tissue of origin for the cyst. Pathologically, it is a foregut cyst.

The embryonic gut forms from the endoderm in the fourth week of development. The foregut is the cephalad portion from which the larynx and trachea bud at the end of the fourth week. The most cephalad portion of the foregut is in proximity to Rathke's pouch.[3] Throughout its length, the foregut is in proximity

Case Ten 61

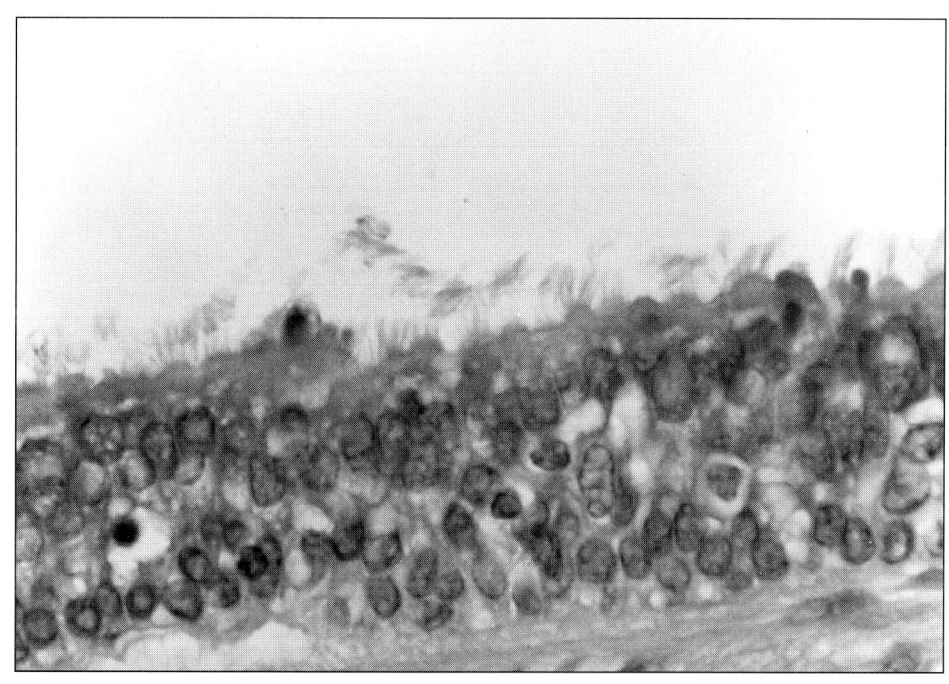

Figure 10–1. Pseudostratified ciliated epithelium lines the surface of some of the cystic structures.

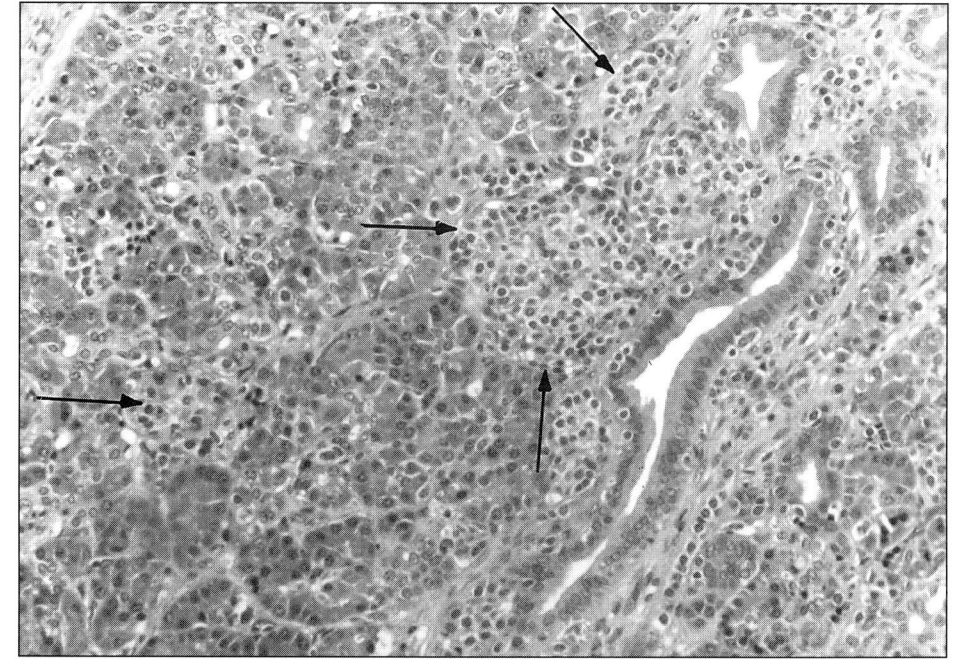

Figure 10–2. Pancreatic tissue, including islet tissue (arrows), is found in many of the sections through this foregut cyst.

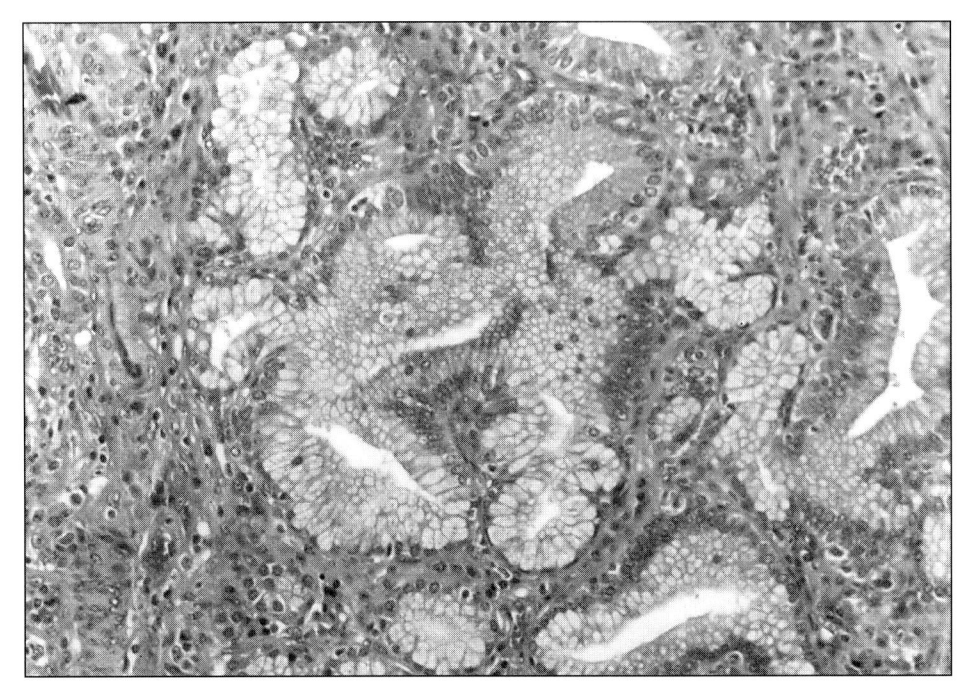

Figure 10–3. Gastric epithelium predominates in most sections of the cyst wall.

to the neural tube. The caudal end of the foregut gives rise to the pancreatic and hepatic buds. Malformations of foregut derivatives can involve the pituitary and hypothalamus, the oropharynx and nasopharynx, the cervical and thoracic spine and spinal cord, the larynx, trachea, bronchi, lungs, esophagus, stomach, proximal duodenum, pancreas, gallbladder, and liver. Duplications and cysts develop from abnormal pouches that emerge and continue to grow from the foregut.[4] An alternative explanation is that recanalization of the solid foregut fails to progress normally, forming two lumens.[3,5] Favara et al advanced the hypothesis that a vascular accident causes necrosis of a segment of gut and that in healing, regenerating tissue forms cysts and duplications.[6] Dehner regards bronchogenic cysts as examples of foregut cysts.[7] Branchial pouch cysts and thyroglossal duct cysts can be placed in this category. Proximity to the neural canal results in communication of the foregut with the spinal canal or spinal cord. Dumbbell-shaped neurenteric cysts sometimes develop with expansions anterior and posterior to the split vertebral bodies. The malformed vertebrae appear as hemivertebrae in radiographs.

Foregut cysts are more common in girls than in boys, especially if the bronchopulmonary tree is involved. Cysts most often occur in the lower end of the thoracic foregut.[7] The diagnosis may be made antenatally with ultrasound examination or at birth, and most cases occur in the first 18 months of extrauterine life. Associated congenital abnormalities include scoliosis and spina bifida.[8] Cardiac anomalies have also been reported.[6,9] Asymptomatic cysts may escape detection until adulthood.

Complications of thoracic cysts are related to respiratory difficulty[10] and swallowing problems.[8,11] Distal or infradiaphragmatic foregut cysts may present as a mass or extend through a defect in the diaphragm into the thoracic cavity where they may be tethered to vertebrae.[6] They usually lie in the right hemithorax. If fistulae develop with the bronchial tree, a bronchopulmonary foregut cyst is the result. Gastric mucosa is the predominant cell type, but ciliated epithelium, neural tissue, and pancreatic tissue are also seen with fair frequency.[8,12] An adrenal rest has been reported in the wall of a foregut cyst.[13] If the foregut cyst contains gastric epithelium, peptic ulcers may form and can bleed or perforate into the chest cavity, pericardium, or lung. Burgner et al described such a case in a neonate with hemoptysis and respiratory distress.[14] Adenocarcinomas have developed in thoracic cysts of foregut origin,[15] one 39 years after the cyst was first discovered.[16]

Foregut derivatives form other structural abnormalities such as laryngeal or tracheal stenosis. Davis et al reported a solid cartilaginous sleeve of the trachea in one child who also had craniosynostosis.[17] The tracheal cartilages and smooth muscle coats of the foregut derivatives are derived from the splanchnic mesoderm surrounding the primitive foregut. Foregut cysts of the tongue with intestinal,[6] respiratory, and squamous epithelium have caused feeding difficulty in neonates.[18] Because of the foregut's craniad proximity to Rathke's pouch and the developing brain, some authorities believe colloid cysts of the cerebral ventricles are foregut derivatives.[19] Mackenzie and Gilbert found cuboidal and columnar epithelium with mucus-containing goblet cells and cilia in a colloid cyst. Stains for cytokeratin, epithelial membrane antigen, and carcinoembryonic antigen were positive, while stains for vimentin and glial fibrillary acidic protein were negative.[19] At the caudal end of the foregut, hepatic or pancreatic cysts may form from foregut derivatives. Ciliated epithelium is the diagnostic feature that distinguishes origin of these cysts from that of the foregut.[20-22]

Midgut and hindgut duplications and cysts are far more numerous than foregut cysts.[8] These more caudal lesions usually have fewer complications than do foregut malformations.[23,24]

Subsequent information: The patient had a fourth operation to correct a hiatal hernia. She has not grown well but is otherwise in reasonably good health at 6 years of age.

DIAGNOSIS: Foregut cyst

References

1. Dahms BB. The gastrointestinal tract. In: Stocker JT, Dehner LP, eds. *Pediatric Pathology*. Philadelphia: JB Lippincott Co; 1992:655.
2. Reed JC, Sobonya RE. Morphologic analysis of foregut cysts in the thorax. *Am J Roentgen Rad Ther Nucl Med* 1974;120:851–860.
3. Hamilton WJ, Mossman HW. *Human Embryology-Prenatal Development of Form and Function*. 4th ed. Baltimore: Williams & Wilkins Co; 1972:292.
4. Veeneklaas GMH. Pathogenesis of intrathoracic gastrogenic cysts. *Am J Dis Child* 1952;83:500–507.

5. Moore KL. *The Developing Human: Clinically Oriented Embryology.* 2nd ed. Philadelphia: WB Saunders Co; 1977:188–220.
6. Favara BE, Franciosi RA, Akers DR. Enteric duplications: Thirty-seven cases—A vascular theory of pathogenesis. *Am J Dis Child* 1971;122:501–506.
7. Dehner LP. *Pediatric Surgical Pathology.* 2nd ed. Baltimore: Williams & Wilkins; 1987:334.
8. Carachi R, Burgner DP. Thoracic foregut duplications. *Arch Dis Child* 1994;71:395–396.
9. Ildstad ST, Tollerud DJ, Weiss RG, Ryan DP, McGowan MA, Martin MW. Duplications of the alimentary tract: Clinical characteristics, preferred treatment and associated malformations. *Ann Surg* 1988;208:184–189.
10. Citardi MJ, Taquina DN, Eisen R. Primitive foregut cysts: A cause of airway obstruction in the newborn. *Otolaryngol Head Neck Surg* 1994;111:533–537.
11. Kirwan WO, Walbaum PR, McCormack RJM. Cystic intrathoracic derivatives of the foregut and their complications. *Thorax* 1973;28:424–428.
12. Macpherson RI. Gastrointestinal tract duplications: Clinical, pathologic, etiologic, and radiologic considerations. *Radiographics* 1993;13:1063–1080.
13. Wright JR Jr, Gillis DA. Mediastinal foregut cyst containing an intramural adrenal cortical rest: A case report and review of supradiaphragmatic adrenal rests. *Pediatr Pathol* 1993;13:401–407.
14. Burgner DP, Carachi R, Beattie TJ. Foregut duplication cyst presenting as neonatal respiratory distress and haemoptysis. *Thorax* 1994;49:287–288.
15. Chuang MT, Barba FA, Kaneko M, Tierstein AS. Adenocarcinoma arising in an intrathoracic duplication of foregut origin: A case report and review of the literature. *Cancer* 1981;47:1887–1890.
16. Olsen JB, Clemmensen O, Andersen K. Adenocarcinoma arising in a foregut cyst of the mediastinum. *Ann Thorac Surg* 1991;51:497–499.
17. Davis S, Bove KE, Wells TR, Hartsell B, Weinberg A, Gilbert E. Tracheal cartilaginous sleeve. *Pediatr Pathol* 1992;12:349–364.
18. Wiersma R, Hadley GP, Bosenberg AT, Chrystal V. Intralingual cysts of foregut origin. *J Pediatr Surg* 1992;27:1404–1406.
19. Mackenzie IR, Gilbert JJ. Cysts of the neuraxis of endodermal origin. *J Neurol Neurosurg Psychiatr* 1991;54:572–575.
20. Wheeler D, Edmondson HA. Ciliated hepatic foregut cyst. *Am J Surg Pathol* 1984;8:467–470.
21. Terada T, Nakanuma Y, Ohta T, et al. Mucin-histochemical and immunohistochemical profiles of epithelial cells of several types of hepatic cysts. *Virchows Arch A Pathol Anat Histopathol* 1991;419:499–504.
22. Pins MR, Compton CC, Souther JF, Rattner DW. Ciliated enteric duplication cyst presenting as a pancreatic cystic neoplasm: Report of a case with cyst fluid analysis. *Clin Chem* 1992;38:1501–1503.
23. Grosfeld JL, O'Neill JA Jr, Clatworthy HW Jr. Enteric duplication of infancy and childhood: An 18 year review. *Ann Surg* 1970;172:83–90.
24. Salyer DC, Salyer WR, Eggleston JC. Benign developmental cysts of the mediastinum. *Arch Pathol Lab Med* 1977;101:136–139.

Case Eleven

Contributed by Arthur R. Cohen, MD
Charlotte, North Carolina

History

The patient is a 14-year-old girl who presented 12 days before admission with flu-like symptoms including rhinorrhea, intermittent arthralgias, cough, intermittent dizziness, and a low-grade fever. Symptoms abated somewhat, but she experienced fatigue and spiking fevers at night 1 week before admission. Results of a physical examination including the abdomen were normal. Laboratory studies showed mild leukocytosis (15,000) (15×10^9/L) with a left shift. She was thought to have a viral syndrome, and tetracycline was initiated. Three days before admission, she developed diffuse upper abdominal pain, vomiting, and some diarrhea. Right upper quadrant tenderness was detected on physical examination, but neither organomegaly nor masses were palpated. The possibility of cholecystitis was considered. On the day before admission, an ultrasound was performed to exclude cholecystitis, but instead, a solid mass was identified in the right kidney. A separate 1-cm density, in addition to multiple cysts, was present in the same kidney. The contralateral kidney also contained multiple cysts. Further imaging studies disclosed a mass in the right kidney that extended into the retroperitoneum with apparent involvement of contiguous lymph nodes (Figure 11–1). A right nephrectomy was subsequently performed. The patient is almost 1 year postsurgery and is doing well without evidence of local or distant disease. The family history failed to disclose other members with tuberous sclerosis.

Dr Dehner: As noted from the clinical history, this 14-year-old girl had a tumor in the right kidney and the nephrectomy specimen contained a $10 \times 6 \times 7.5$ cm mass at one pole. On cut surface, the mass had a light tan to gray appearance and focal areas of necrosis were noted (Figure 11–2). There was a 2.5-cm cyst adjacent to the mass and several smaller cysts were also identified in the renal parenchyma. A second nodule measuring 1 cm in diameter with a yellowish-gray surface was present approximately 4 cm from the larger mass.

    The dominant tumor mass is a spindle cell neoplasm with extensive areas of necrosis. There are nodular or multinodular and interfascicular patterns of growth associated with this neoplasm (Figure 11–3, top and bottom). The tumor cells have indistinct cell borders and prominent eosinophilic granular to fibrillary cytoplasm. Multiple thick-walled vascular structures blended into the surrounding tumor (Figure 11–4). Some nuclear atypism was present, but mitotic figures were difficult to identify. On the basis of the predominant microscopic appearance of the large mass, the following questions arise: Is this neoplasm primary in the kidney or has it arisen in the retroperitoneum and invaded the kidney?

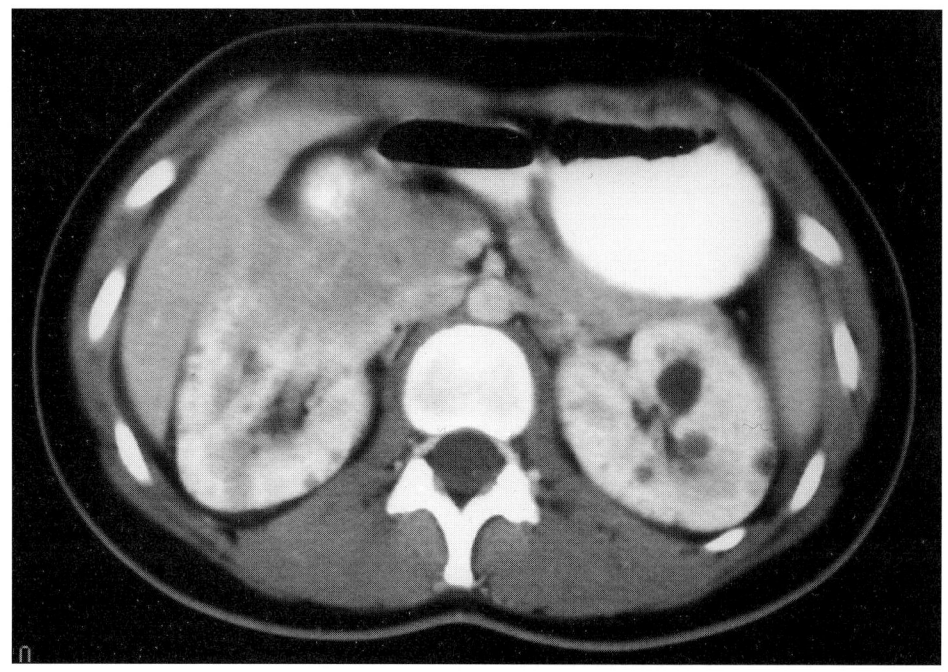

66   *Placental, Neonatal, and Pediatric Pathology*

Figure 11–1. An abdominal computerized tomogram reveals a large, somewhat inhomogeneous mass in the right kidney that has extended directly into the retroperitoneum. Multiple cysts of varying sizes are present in both kidneys.

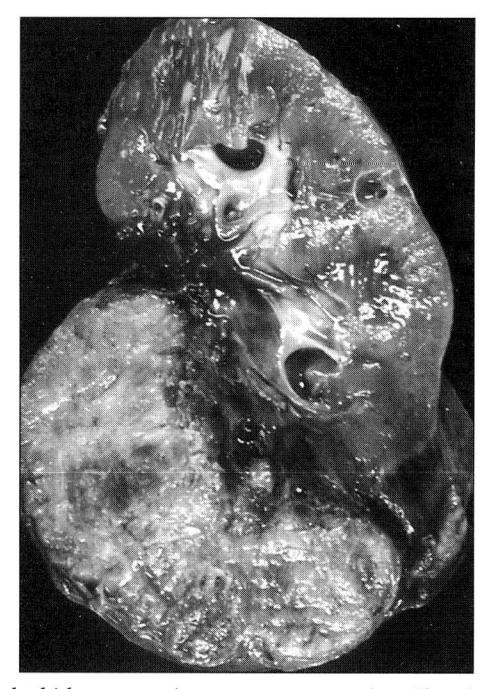

Figure 11–2. The right kidney contains a mass measuring 10 × 6 × 7.5 cm and shows a coarsely nodular surface with areas of necrosis on cross section, which accounts for the irregularity in the density of the mass on computed tomography.

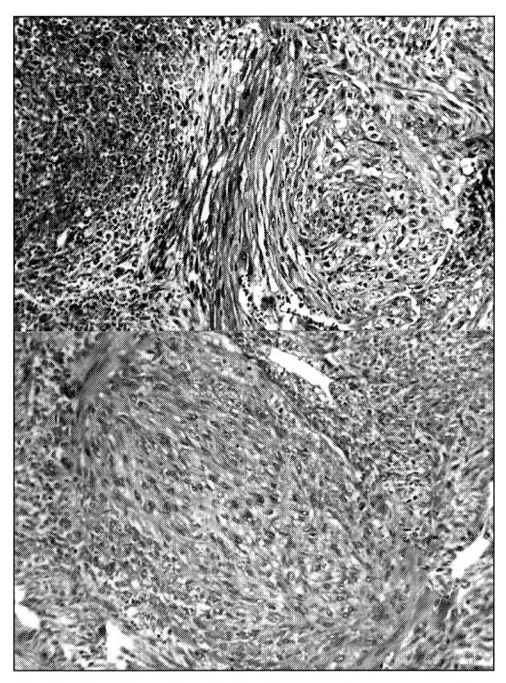

Figure 11–3. Interfascicular (top) and nodular (bottom) patterns alternated as the dominant patterns throughout the tumor. Necrosis is present as interspersed confluent areas (top).

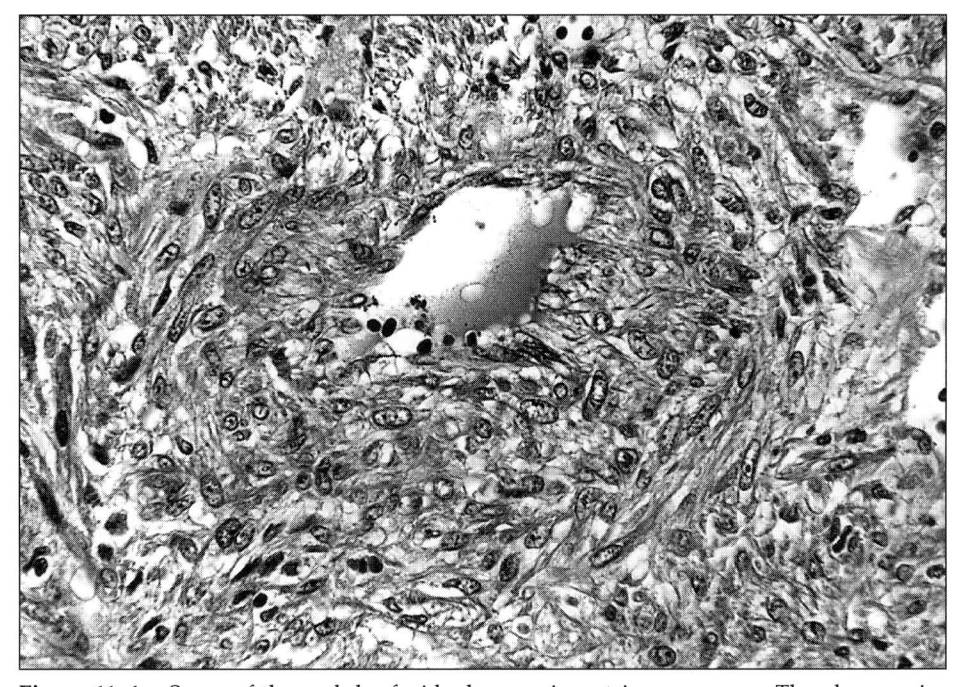

Figure 11–4. Some of the nodular foci had an angiocentric appearance. The plump spindle cells blend into the surrounding tumor cells with similar features.

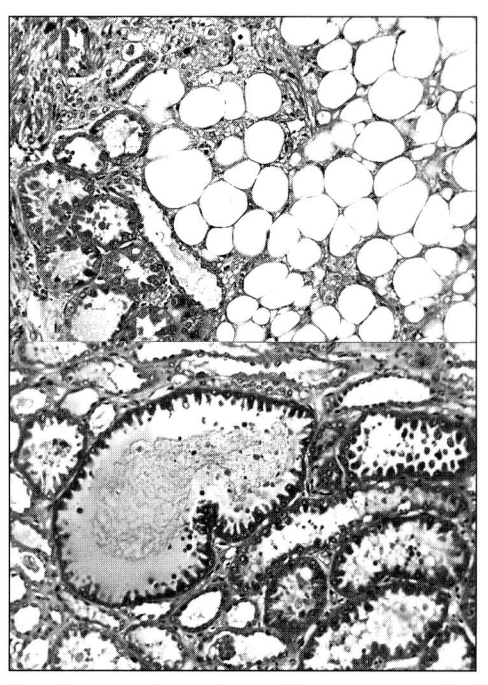

Figure 11–5. Multiple microscopic angiomyolipomas are a feature of the renal parenchyma surrounding the dominant mass (top). Note the hobnail character of the adjacent renal tubular epithelial cells (bottom). Cysts of varying sizes with plump eosinophilic tubular lining cells are present throughout the kidney.

If this tumor is a primary neoplasm of the kidney, does it correspond to any of the more conventional renal tumors of childhood? It is fair to state that this neoplasm does not resemble Wilms' renal tumor or any of the non-Wilms' tumors of childhood. Is this neoplasm, despite the age of the patient, possibly a sarcomatoid variant of renal cell carcinoma? Immunohistochemistry was performed with anticipation about the results since the remainder of the kidney had several microscopic foci of readily identifiable angiomyolipoma and cysts that were lined by oncocytic epithelium with focal hyperplasia of the type associated with tuberous sclerosis (TS) (Figure 11–5, top and bottom). The separate 1-cm nodule represented a renal cell carcinoma with tubular formation with granular cells showing low- to intermediate-grade nuclear abnormalities (Figure 11–6, top and bottom). The angiomyolipomas had directly invaded the hilar lymph nodes (Figure 11–7). There was no evidence of metastasis from the renal cell carcinoma. Immunohistochemically, the spindle cell tumor showed diffuse positivity for smooth muscle actin and HMB-45 (Figure 11–8, top and bottom; Table 11–1). Desmin and muscle-specific actin reactivity was principally confined to the blood vessels.

Postoperatively, further clinical history revealed that the patient had had some seizures in infancy that were apparently associated with fever. An inspection of the malar skin showed the presence of multiple small papular lesions that

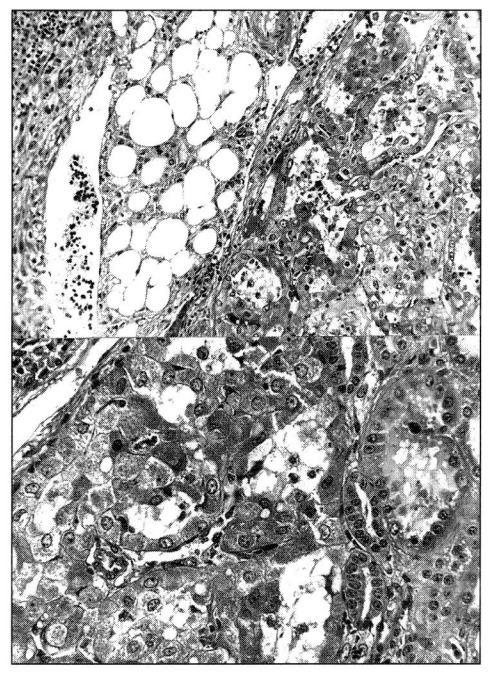

Figure 11–6. The periphery of the renal cell carcinoma abuts a focus of angiomyolipoma (top). A comparison of the granular tumor cells forming the neoplastic tubules (bottom left) can be made with contiguous nonneoplastic tubules (bottom right) with eosinophilic hobnail epithelial cells of the type seen in tuberous sclerosis.

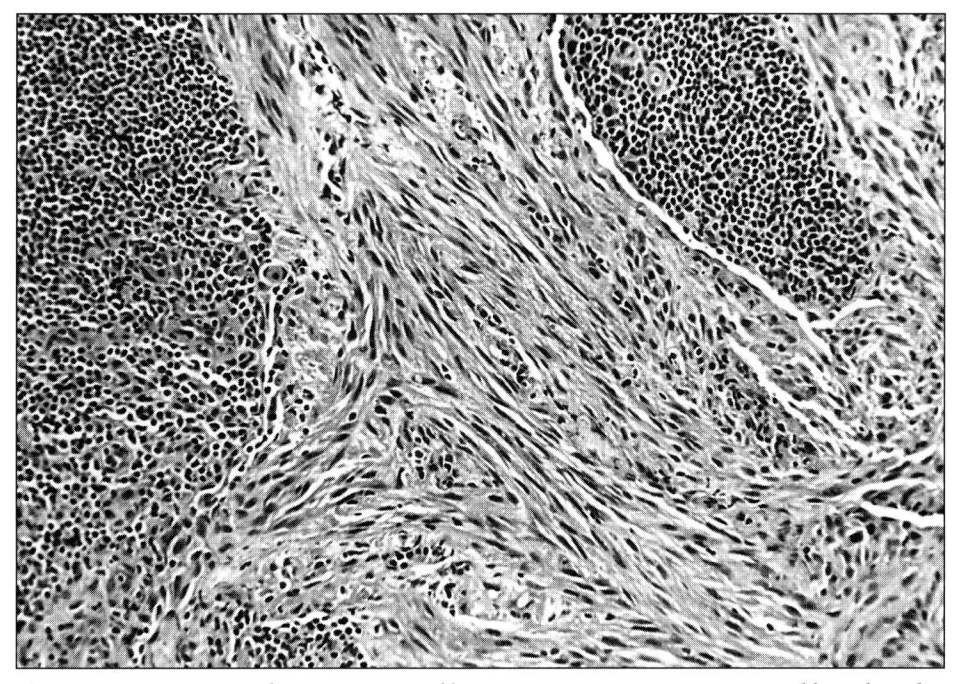

Figure 11–7. Angiomyolipoma is seen infiltrating a contiguous retroperitoneal lymph node.

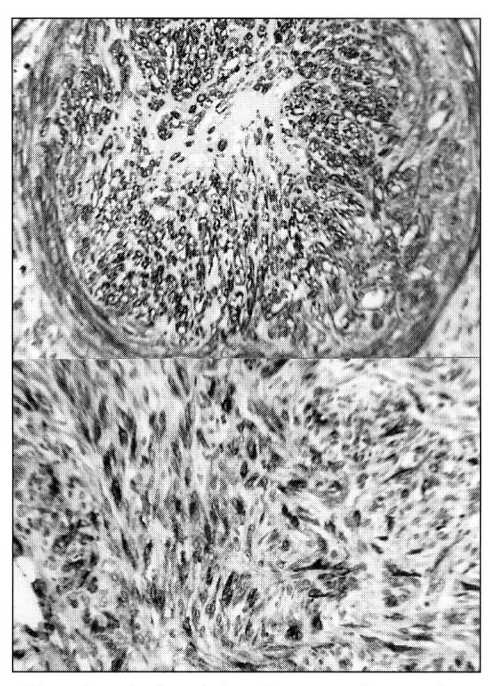

Figure 11–8. Immunohistochemical staining for smooth muscle actin (top) and HMB-45 (bottom) is characteristic of angiomyolipoma.

Table 11–1. Differential Immunohistochemistry of Renal Cell Carcinoma, Smooth Muscle Tumor, Angiomyolipoma, and Peripheral Nerve Sheath Neoplasm

Tumor	VIM	CK	EMA	MSA	DES	S100	HMB45
RCC	±	+	±	–	–	–	–
LM/LMS	+	±	–	+	+	±	–
AML	+	–	–	+	+	–	+
PNSN	+	–	–	–	–	+	–

Abbreviations: RCC = renal cell carcinoma; LM/LMS = leiomyoma-leiomyosarcoma; AML = angiomyolipoma; PNSN = peripheral nerve sheath neoplasm; VIM = vimentin, CK = cytokeratin; EMA = epithelial membrane antigen; MSA = muscle-specific actin; DES = desmin; S100 = S-100 protein.

were regarded as consistent with adenoma sebaceum. An electroencephalogram obtained several months after the nephrectomy failed to depict any seizure activity. Based on the aggregate of clinical and pathologic findings, this patient appears to fulfill the criteria for the diagnosis of TS.[1]

Angiomyolipoma (AML) is a well-recognized tumor of the kidney that has also been reported in extrarenal sites including the perinephric and retroperitoneal soft tissues, liver, skin, spleen, and uterus.[2–4] There are still some uncertainties whether to consider an AML as a hamartoma or a true neoplasm. Arguments in favor of its neoplastic nature include rare instances of malignant transformation and the ability of AML to grow locally into regional lymph nodes (as in this case), the renal vein, and the inferior vena cava.[5] The association between TS and AML is well documented, but there are other renal manifestations of TS.[6–11] One or more renal lesions of TS were present in almost 50% of affected patients in one clinical series, but AMLs of the kidney were noted with some frequency at autopsy (67% of individuals with TS), which reflects the fact that these lesions may remain as asymptomatic foci.[6,11] Tubular cysts are the most common abnormalities of the kidney in TS,[10] whereas renal cell carcinoma is one of the least frequent findings, with an estimated incidence of 1% to 3% of cases.[12–14]

What percentage of patients with AML have TS? This figure tends to vary from one series to another. For instance, Steiner and associates noted that 17% of patients in their study of 35 individuals with AML had TS.[15] It is generally acknowledged that most patients with AML do not have TS.[3] The sporadic AML typically presents in a middle-age woman with a unilateral mass. Some clinical and pathologic clues that an AML is a manifestation of TS include the following features: young age at presentation (less than 40 years old, which makes a case in childhood especially suspect); a large tumor (greater than 4 cm, likewise making our case at 10 cm very suspect); spontaneous hemorrhage (a complication of the larger AMLs); and multiplicity of lesions in the kidney with infiltrating borders, calcified spicules, and tuberous inclusions.[8,9,16–18] Bilateral AMLs are present in approximately 80% of individuals with TS, whereas most sporadic AMLs are unilateral.[3] When a renal cell carcinoma presents in a child, the possibility of TS should be given some consideration.

As the designation of AML implies, the tumor is composed of three tissue components: blood vessels, smooth muscle, and fat; but these various tissues are not necessarily represented equally in a given tumor, as our case illustrates. Many of the microscopic foci of AML in the surrounding kidney in our case demonstrated the classic triphasic features to better advantage. When an AML is composed almost exclusively of adipose tissue with atypical nuclear features, the diagnosis of well-differentiated or lipoma-like liposarcoma may become the preferred interpretation (Figure 11–9, top and bottom). Despite the fact that a single differentiated tissue may be dominant in a particular AML, it is generally the rule that the other two components are represented elsewhere in the tumor as microscopic foci. The smooth muscle of the AML and lymphoangiomyomatosis have the unique immunohistochemical attribute of expressing the melanocytic marker, MBH-45.[19–21] An initial diagnostic dilemma in our case of an apparent angiomyomatous neoplasm was resolved in favor of an AML with the unequivocal expression of HMB-45.

Tuberous sclerosis is one of the neurophakomatoses and like the other disorders in this group of congenital hamartomatoses, it is an autosomal dominant disorder.[22,23] The spontaneous mutation rate varies from 66% to 80%, and the prevalence is one case per 6000 to 9000 individuals.[22] There are a number of phenotypic manifestations of TS that have been categorized as primary, secondary, and tertiary features by Roach et al.[1] Angiomyolipoma and cysts of the kidney are secondary manifestations, whereas facial angiofibromas (the so-called ade-

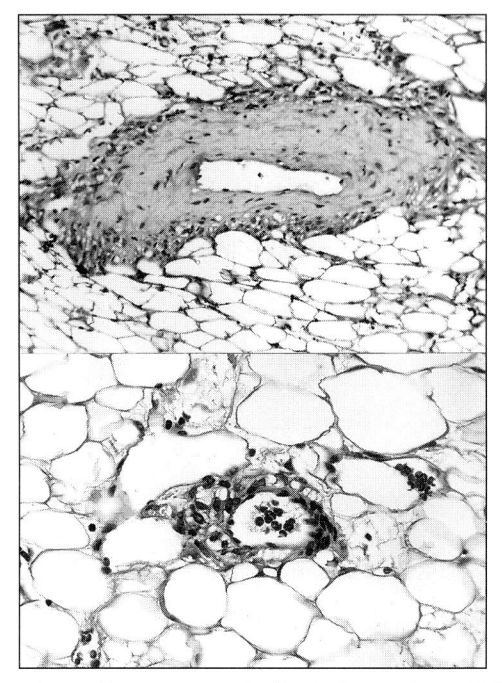

Figure 11–9. This angiomyolipoma arose in the kidney of a middle-aged woman who presented with flank pain. Adipose tissue with some atypical features posed the possibility of liposarcoma; however, the hyalinized blood vessels (top) and small vessels with an incomplete cuff of myogenic cells (bottom) are features of an angiomyolipoma.

noma sebaceum), subungual fibromas, cortical tubers, subependymal giant cell astrocytoma, and multiple retinal astrocytomas are primary features. A rare presentation of TS is bilateral cystic renal disease, which may resemble adult polycystic kidney disease (ADPKD), which is interesting in light of the fact that one of the two genetic loci identified in TS is on chromosome 16 (16p13), which is also one of the loci of ADPKD.[24-28] The other gene locus in TS is present on chromosome 9 (9q34).[25] A translocation, t(3;12)(p26.3;q23.3), has been reported in a child with TS.[28] Tuberous sclerosis appears to be a genetically heterogeneous condition since a third locus may exist as well.

DIAGNOSIS: Angiomyolipoma, renal cell carcinoma, and multiple cysts of the kidney

References

1. Roach ES, Smith M, Huttenlocher P, et al. Report of the Diagnostic Criteria Committee of the National Tuberous Sclerosis Association. *J Child Neurol* 1992;7:221–224.
2. Blute ML, Malek RS, Segura JEW. Angiomyolipoma: Clinical metamorphosis and concepts for management. *J Urol* 1988;139:20–24.

3. Murphy WM, Beckwith JB, Farrow GM. *Tumors of the Kidney, Bladder, and Related Urinary Structures.* Washington, DC: Armed Forces Institute of Pathology; 1994:161–174.
4. Peh WC, Lim BH, Tam PC. Case report: Perinephric angiomyolipomas in tuberous sclerosis. *Br J Urol* 1994;67:1026–1029.
5. Taylor RS, Joseph DB, Kohaut EC, et al. Renal angiomyolipoma associated with lymph node involvement and renal cell carcinoma in patients with tuberous sclerosis. *J Urol* 1989;141:930–932.
6. Zimmerhackl LB, Rehm M, Kaufmehl K, et al. Renal involvement in tuberous sclerosis complex: A retrospective survey. *Pediatr Nephrol* 1994;8:451–457.
7. Bernstein J, Robbins TO, Kissane JM. The renal lesions of tuberous sclerosis. *Semin Diagn Pathol* 1986;3:97–105.
8. Stillwell TJ, Gomer MR, Kelalis PP. Renal lesions in tuberous sclerosis. *J Urol* 1987;138:477–481.
9. Bernstein J, Robbins TO. Renal involvement in tuberous sclerosis. *Ann NY Acad Sci* 1991;615:36–49.
10. Torres VE, King BF, Holley KE, et al. The kidney in the tuberous sclerosis complex. *Adv Nephrol* 1994;23:43–70.
11. Robbins TO, Bernstein J. Renal involvement. In: Gomez MR, ed. *Tuberous Sclerosis.* 2nd ed. New York: Raven Press; 1988:133–146.
12. Weinblatt ME, Kahn E, Kochen J. Renal cell carcinoma in patients with tuberous sclerosis. *Pediatrics* 1987; 80:898–903.
13. Ueda J, Kobayashi Y, Itoh H, Itatani H. Angiomyolipoma and renal cell carcinoma occurring in same kidney: CT evaluation. *J Comput Assist Tomogr* 1987;11:340–341.
14. Graves N, Barnes WF. Renal cell carcinoma and angiomyolipoma in tuberous sclerosis: Case report. *J Urol* 1986;135:122–123.
15. Steiner MS, Goldman SM, Fishman EK, Marshall FF. The natural history of renal angiomyolipomas. *J Urol* 1993;150:1782–1786.
16. Van Baal JG, Becker AC, Fleury P, Brummelkamp WH. Renal angiomyolipomas: Could histology serve as a marker of tuberous sclerosis? *Histopathology* 1990;17:180–182.
17. Azmy AF, Stephenson J, Ziervogel M. Angiomyolipomas causing life-threatening hematuria in a child with tuberous sclerosis. *J Pediatr Surg* 1989;24: 1308–1309.
18. Van Baal JG, Smits NJ, Keeman JN, et al. The evolution of renal angiomyolipomas in patients with tuberous sclerosis. *J Urol* 1994;152:35–38.
19. Ashfaq R, Weinberg AG, Albores-Saavedra J. Renal angiomyolipomas and HMB-45 reactivity. *Cancer* 1993;71:3091–3097.
20. Sturtz CL, Dabbs DJ. Angiomyolipomas: The nature and expression of the HMB45 antigen. *Mod Pathol* 1994;7:842–845.
21. Chan JK, Tsang WY, Pau MY, et al. Lymphangiomyomatosis and angiolipoma: Closely related entities characterized by hamartomatous proliferation of HMB45-positive smooth muscle. *Histopathology* 1993;22:445–455.
22. Berg RO. Neurocutaneous syndromes: Phakomatoses and allied conditions. In: Swaim KF, ed. *Neurology: Principles and Practice.* St Louis: Mosby; 1994:1045–1069.

23. Roach ES, Delgado MR. Tuberous sclerosis. *Dermatol Clin* 1995;13:157–161.
24. Campos A, Figueroa ET, Gunasekaran S, Garin EH. Early presentation of tuberous sclerosis as bilateral renal cysts. *J Urol* 1993;149:1077–1079.
25. Povey S, Burley MW, Attwood J, et al. Two loci for tuberous sclerosis: One on 9q34 and one on 16p13. *Ann Hum Genet* 1994;58:107–127.
26. European Chromosome 16 Tuberous Sclerosis Consortium. Identification and characterization of the tuberous sclerosis gene on chromosome 16. *Cell* 1993;75:1305–1315.
27. The International Polycystic Kidney Disease Consortium. Polycystic kidney disease: The complete structure of the PKD1 gene and its protein. *Cell* 1995;81:289–298.
28. Fahsold R, Rott HD, Claussen U, Schmalenberger B. Tuberous sclerosis in a child with de novo translocation (t(3;12)(p26.3;q23.3). *Clin Genet* 1991;40: 326–328.

Case Twelve

Contributed by Louis P. Dehner, MD
St Louis, Missouri

History

The patient is a 7-month-old boy whose father (a physician) detected an abdominal mass. A large mass replaced the right kidney, and several smaller masses were identified in the left kidney (Figure 12–1). A right nephrectomy was subsequently performed. He continues to do well 20 months after the initial diagnosis.

Dr Dehner: After it was discovered that this infant had bilateral renal masses and a dominant mass in the right kidney, open biopsies of both kidneys were performed to decide on the appropriate therapy based on the interpretation of these specimens. The biopsy of the large right renal mass revealed a Wilms' tumor with nests of primitive blastema surrounded by a loose spindle cell stroma (Figure 12–2, top and bottom). Biopsy results of the contralateral kidney disclosed nephroblastic proliferations with somewhat different microscopic features from a classic Wilms' tumor. There were individual primitive blastemal nests, immature tubules intermixed among more normal-appearing tubules, and an immature spindle cell stroma (Figure 12–3, top and bottom). Occasional dilated cysts were also present. The impression was that these immature structures had either infiltrated into otherwise normal kidney or that there was dissynchronous maturation of the renal tubules; these histologic features are characteristic of intralobar nephroblastomatosis, one of the progenitor lesions of Wilms' tumor.[1] Preoperative chemotherapy was administered to this infant; thus the explanation for the perplexing appearance of this Wilms' tumor. Grossly, the right kidney weighed 760 g. The upper and midportion of the kidney was occupied by a well-circumscribed mass measuring 12 × 10 × 9 cm. On cut surface, the mass had a gray to pinkish-tan appearance with a network of white fibrous strands (Figure 12–4, top and bottom). Along the lateral aspect of the dominant mass, a smaller nodule measuring 5.5 × 4.5 × 5 cm with a necrotic, brownish-green appearance was noted. Sections of the right kidney disclosed remarkably innocuous histologic findings, consisting of a bland, relatively hypocellular fibrous stroma, foci of differentiated skeletal muscle, and isolated glomeruli and tubules (Figure 12–5, top and bottom). There are also scattered foci of perilobar and intralobar nephrogenic rests. Residual Wilms' tumor was not identified after extensive sampling of the mass.

Preoperative chemotherapy is commonly used in the management of some solid malignant neoplasms of childhood, including osteosarcoma and Ewing's sarcoma. The pathologic examination of the resected specimen in these cases is directed toward the semiquantitative assessment of tumor necrosis as a measure

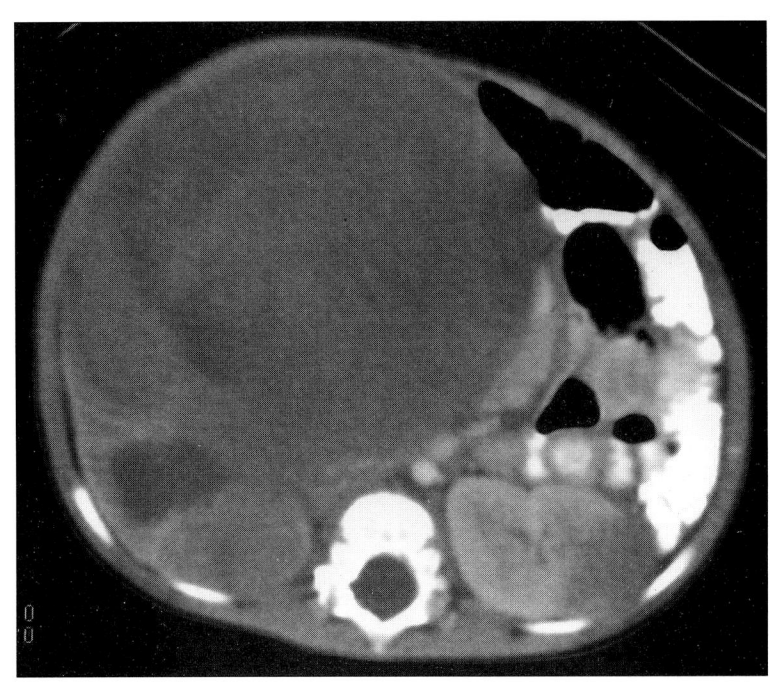

Figure 12–1. Computed tomography scan demonstrates a large mass and a second smaller contiguous mass in the right kidney and a small mass in the left kidney.

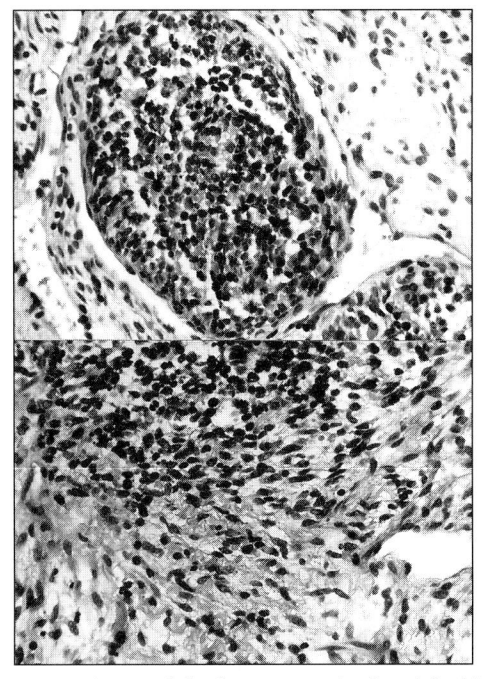

Figure 12–2. The biopsy specimen of the large mass in the right kidney shows a nodule of blastema (top) and immature skeletal muscle (bottom), which are features of classic Wilms' tumor.

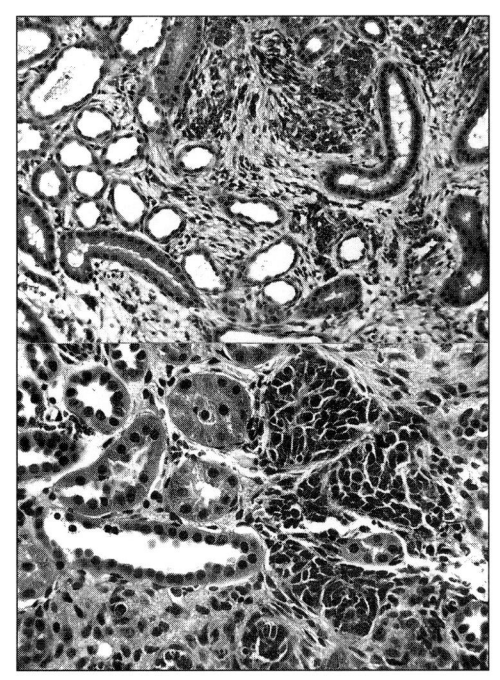

Figure 12–3. A biopsy specimen of the left kidney discloses a nephroblastic proliferation with an intermixture of immature stroma with a spectrum of tubular abnormalities (top) and small blastematous nests adjacent to more normal-appearing tubules (bottom). These are the histologic features of an intralobar nephrogenic rest.

of response to chemotherapy. In the case of other solid malignant neoplasms, the decision to administer preoperative chemotherapy is based on the inability to primarily resect the tumor; the goal of chemotherapy in these cases is to effect reduction in tumor size so that a complete resection can be accomplished. A biopsy of the tumor is performed before chemotherapy as a rule in these cases, but the tumor sample is usually small and for that reason, it may be difficult to evaluate the neoplasm for purposes of pathologic grading. For instance, it is impossible in our case to know whether anaplasia was present or not. There is the occasional case in which the biopsy specimen is so small or distorted by crush artifact that a pathologic diagnosis is impossible.

The systematic documentation of the morphologic effects of preoperative chemotherapy on various types of pediatric neoplasms is limited in the literature. Zuppan et al[2] reviewed the experience of the National Wilms' Tumor Study (NWTS) and identified 140 (5.6%) cases from a total of 2489 Wilms' tumors that had received preoperative chemotherapy. In the United States, preoperative chemotherapy has not been a common practice, but in European countries a substantial proportion of Wilms' tumors are managed in this fashion. One can anticipate some of the problems, including the inability to accurately stage the tumor, and in some cases, the renal neoplasm may not be a Wilms' tumor at all. On occasion, a prechemotherapy biopsy specimen may not have been obtained since the clinical and imaging studies were judged to be typical of Wilms' tumor.

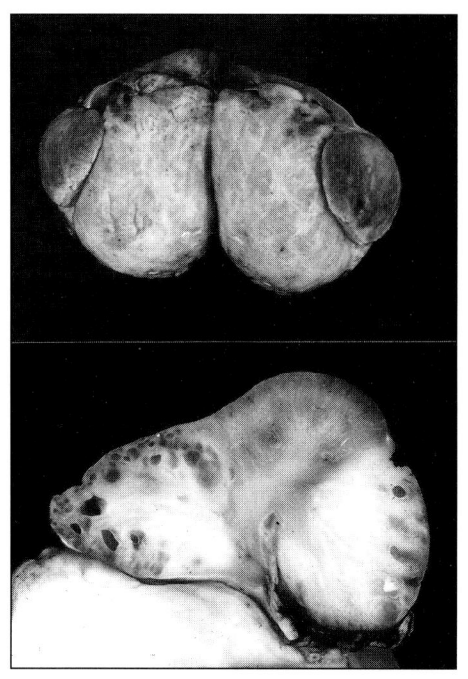

Figure 12–4. The right kidney is largely replaced by a white circumscribed mass with an adjacent darker nodule. The larger mass has a pale tan appearance that is interrupted by a network of white fibrous strands (top). Additional sectioning of the kidney revealed two separate nodules representing hyperplastic nephrogenic rests as other manifestations of nephroblastomatosis (bottom).

An earlier study by Bannayan et al[3] reported that preoperative irradiation to Wilms' tumors produced a "maturational" effect. The histologic characteristics in our case would imply that there had been a considerable chemotherapeutic effect with total ablation of the blastomatous components that were present in the biopsy specimen. Benign-appearing fibrous tissue and loosely arranged spindle cells, isolated atrophic tubules, and small islands of tubules and cysts with intracystic papillary structures and maturing skeletal muscle were the residual tissues identified in the present case. Adjacent to the large mass there were smaller nodules representing additional foci of nephroblastomatosis (see Figure 12–4, bottom). This so-called maturational effect of chemotherapy or radiation therapy has been observed in metastases of Wilms' tumor and in malignant germ cell tumors with only residual mature teratomatous elements. Saxena et al[4] have questioned whether maturation also occurs in pretreated hepatoblastomas, which was evident by the presence of osteoid after chemotherapy; osteoid was seen infrequently in those hepatoblastomas that had been primarily resected. Chemotherapy and irradiation may induce maturation, but it could be argued that the chemo- or radiation-sensitive components are seemingly the highly proliferative primitive or blastomatous population of cells that are ablated and only the connective tissue stroma and/or differentiated structures with their low pro-

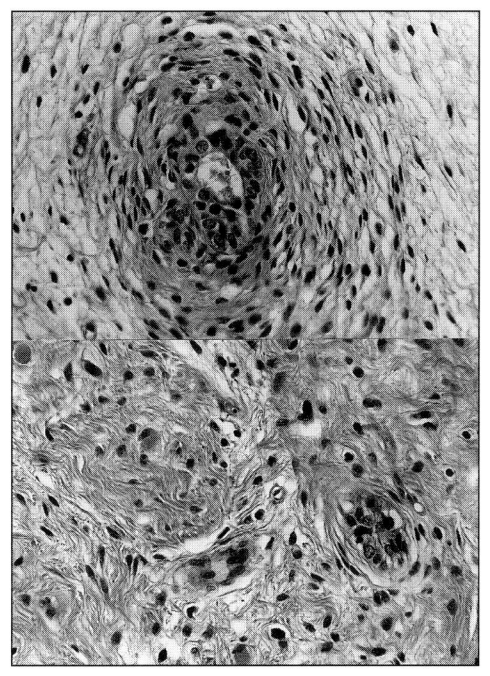

Figure 12–5. Residual structures in the posttreatment Wilms' tumor include small tubules surrounded by a spindle cell stroma resembling the tubules in renal dysplasia (top). Note the presence of the bland, somewhat immature-appearing mesenchyme (top) and the equally innocuous fibrous stroma (bottom), which together were the dominant tissues in the tumor.

liferative index remain as the residual elements since they are unlikely to be affected by cell cycle–interrupting agents (Table 12–1).

Several years ago, this child would have been regarded as having bilateral Wilms' tumors; however, the concepts developed by Beckwith and colleagues[1] over the past 15 years have provided us with a better understanding of the histogenesis of Wilms' tumor from its inception in progenitor lesions including perilobar and intralobar nephrogenic rests and hyperplastic and adenomatous rests.[5] These histogenetic concepts have been wedded to the molecular events in the normal development of the kidney and the formation of Wilms' tumor.[6,7]

Wilms' tumor is the most common primary malignant neoplasm of the kidney in childhood (Table 12–2).[5,8] It was thought at one time that all primary renal neoplasms in children were Wilms' tumors or variants thereof. For instance, a pure spindle variant of Wilms' tumor was recognized as a neoplasm of infancy, unlike most Wilms' tumors, which are diagnosed in children between the ages of 1 and 5 years; this spindle cell variant of Wilms' tumor was known to have an excellent prognosis unlike most other Wilms' tumors and is now recognized as the mesoblastic nephroma.[5,8,9] There were also other renal neoplasms in children that did not have the classic triphasic features of Wilms' tumor but had a monotonous histologic appearance and were considered "sarcomatous" variants of

Table 12–1. Altered Pathologic Features of Some Pediatric Neoplasms After Preoperative Chemotherapy

Tumor Type	Postchemotherapy Histologic Features
Wilms' tumor	Fibromyomatous stroma, skeletal muscle and tubular rests
Neuroblastoma	Neuromatous stroma, differentiated neuroblasts and ganglion cells
Hepatoblastoma	Mature cords of hepatocytes, bile ducts
Rhabdomyosarcoma	Differentiated rhabdomyoblasts or rhabdomyocytes
Mixed malignant germ cell tumor	Mature teratoma and/or dense fibrosis and macrophages
Osteosarcoma	Dense hypocellular fibrous stroma devoid of malignant mesenchymal cells and pale-staining osteoid

Table 12–2. Wilms' Tumor and Other Renal Neoplasms of Childhood*

Tumor Type	Frequency (%)
Classic Wilms' tumor (3%-4% anaplasia) (5%-7% bilateral)	85
Mesoblastic nephroma	5
Clear-cell sarcoma	4
Malignant rhabdoid tumor	2
Others (malignant lymphoma, renal cell carcinoma, and angiomyolipoma)	4
Total	100

*Adapted from Beckwith.[5]

Wilms' tumor; these two tumor types are known presently as the malignant rhabdoid tumor (MRT) and clear-cell sarcoma of the kidney (CCSK).[10–12] In the past, the necessity to histologically grade a Wilms' tumor was nonexistent since the prognosis was universally poor regardless of the microscopic features.[13] As combined modality treatment altered the prognosis in a positive fashion, subsets of tumors emerged with definable and repetitive favorable and unfavorable pathologic features. A classic Wilms' tumor is unfavorable only on the basis of cellular anaplasia as defined by the presence of large, bizarre cells with atypical mitotic figures; this change is either focal or diffuse on the basis of the number of microscopic fields with anaplastic cells.[5] Only 3% to 5% of Wilms' tumors have cellular anaplasia, but effective adjuvant therapy has diminished the unfavorable effect of focal anaplasia on prognosis.[1,8,11] Clear-cell sarcoma of the kidney and MRT account for 4% and 2% to 3%, respectively, of childhood renal neoplasms[5]; both of these tumors are prognostically unfavorable. Aggressive therapy of CCSK regardless of the pathologic stage has resulted in improved survival, which has not been the case with MRT.

Table 12–3. Anomalies and Wilms' Tumor

Anomaly	Frequency(%)
Cryptorchidism	2.8
Hypospadias	1.8
Hemihypertrophy	2.5
Aniridia	1
Beckwith-Wiedemann syndrome	<1
Denys-Drash syndrome	<1

This patient illustrates some of the unique aspects of Wilms' tumor when it presents in a child under 1 year of age. These patients are more likely to have bilateral involvement of the kidneys by precursor lesions, producing the phenomenon known as nephroblastomatosis, which is defined by the presence of "diffuse or multifocal . . . nephrogenic rests or their recognized derivatives. This term applies also to cases where the prior presence of rests can be inferred (eg, multicentric and bilateral Wilms' tumors)."[1] Under the terms of the latter definition, bilaterality of nephroblastomatous lesions in the form of Wilms' tumor on the right side with residual nephrogenic rests in the resected kidney and the contralateral nephrogenic rests indicate that this child has nephroblastomatosis.[1,14] A child with nephroblastomatosis is more likely to have one of the syndromic associations like the Beckwith-Wiedemann syndrome (BWS) or aniridia (Table 12–3). An accompanying syndrome is present in only 1% to 3% of all children with Wilms' tumor. To date, there is no evidence of BWS in this patient.

DIAGNOSIS: Wilms' tumor of the kidney with postchemotherapy changes and bilateral nephroblastomatosis

References

1. Beckwith JB, Kiviat NB, Bonadio JF. Nephrogenic rests, nephroblastomatosis, and the pathogenesis of Wilms' tumor. *Pediatr Pathol* 1990;10:1–36.
2. Zuppan CW, Beckwith JB, Weeks DA, et al. The effect of preoperative therapy on the histologic features of Wilms' tumor. *Cancer* 1991;68:385–394.
3. Bannayan GA, Huvos AG, D'Angio GJ. Effect of irradiation on the maturation of Wilms' tumor. *Cancer* 1971;27:812–818.
4. Saxena R, Leake JL, Shafford EA, et al. Chemotherapy effects on hepatoblastoma: A histologic study. *Am J Surg Pathol* 1993;17:1266–1271.
5. Beckwith JB. Renal neoplasms of childhood. In: Sternberg SS, ed. *Diagnostic Surgical Pathology*. 2nd ed. New York: Raven Press; 1994:1741–1766.
6. Coppes MJ, Haber DA, Girundy PE. Genetic events in the development of Wilms tumor. *N Engl J Med* 1994;331:586–590.
7. Coppes MJ, Campbell CE, Williams BRG. *Wilms' Tumor: Clinical and Morphologic Characterization*. Austin, TX: RG Lander Co; 1995.
8. Kissane JM, Dehner LP. Renal tumors and tumor-like lesions in pediatric patients. *Pediatr Nephrol* 1992;6:365–382.

9. Breslow N, Beckwith JB, Ciol M, Sharples K. Age distribution of Wilms' tumor: Report from the National Wilms' Tumor Study. *Cancer Res* 1988;48:1653–1657.
10. Mireau GW, Beckwith JB, Weeks DA. Ultrastructure and histogenesis of the renal tumors of childhood: An overview. *Ultrastruct Pathol* 1987;11:313–333.
11. Webber BL, Parham DM, Drake LG, Wilimas JA. Renal tumors in childhood. *Pathol Annu* 1992;27(Pt 1):91–132.
12. White KS, Grossman H. Wilms' and associated renal tumors of childhood. *Pediatr Radiol* 1991;21:81–88.
13. Green DM, D'Angio GJ, Beckwith JB, et al. Wilms' tumor (nephroblastoma, renal embryoma). In: Pizzo PA, Poplack DG, eds. *Principles and Practice of Pediatric Oncology.* 2nd ed. Philadelphia: JB Lippincott Co; 1993:713–738.
14. Hennigar RA, Othersen HB Jr, Garvin AJ. Clinicopathologic features of nephroblastomatosis. *Urology* 1989;33:259–270.

Case Thirteen

Contributed by Don B. Singer, MD
Providence, Rhode Island

History

This pregnancy was complicated by oligohydramnios and premature delivery at 30 weeks. The baby's abdomen was massively enlarged, severe respiratory distress was present, and the baby died at 2 hours of age.

Dr Singer: Macroscopically, the kidneys were massive, making up almost one-fourth of the baby's total body weight (Figure 13–1). The kidneys together weighed 630 g and the baby weighed 2710 g. The normal expected weight for both kidneys at 30 weeks' gestation is about 15 g. Although the kidneys were huge, they retained a reniform shape. The liver was more than twice its expected weight and the lungs were hypoplastic, weighing half of what they should. The weights of the remaining organs were within the expected range for the gestational age of the baby.

Microscopically the kidney has innumerable fusiform cysts of the tubules in the upper cortex and more rounded cysts in the deeper cortex and medulla (Figure 13–2). At first glance these features suggest the diagnosis of infantile polycystic kidneys or autosomal recessive polycystic kidney disease (ARPKD). However, in that condition, cysts are limited to the collecting ducts and spare the nephronic tubules and glomeruli. In this case, the cysts involve convoluted tubules, Henle's loops, and collecting ducts. Although sparse, glomerular cysts are also present (Figure 13–3). Intact renal tissue is reduced between the cystic spaces. Deep cortical tubules and collecting ducts have fibromuscular collars and are separated by moderately increased loose, but not quite immature, mesenchymatous, collagenous tissue. No cartilage is present. The liver has hyperplastic portal bile ducts that are elongated and tend to wrap around the outer edges of the portal connective tissue. The ducts are not dilated; rather, they consist of potential cysts. The pancreas has subtle dilatation of the ducts (Figure 13–4). The lungs, in addition to being small, have rounded canalicular and glandular airspaces, many of which are filled with fibrin. Cartilage-containing bronchi are situated within 0.1 mm of the pleural surface, a feature associated with arrest of acinar development in midgestation. In this case, the upward pressure on the diaphragm by the massive kidneys compressed the thoracic spaces and crowded the lungs.

No analysis of renal cystic disease would be complete without mention of experimental models, none of which quite replicate the disease previously described or those to be discussed. Animal models include newborn rats given diphenylamine[1]; newborn Syrian hamsters injected with adrenal corticosteroids,

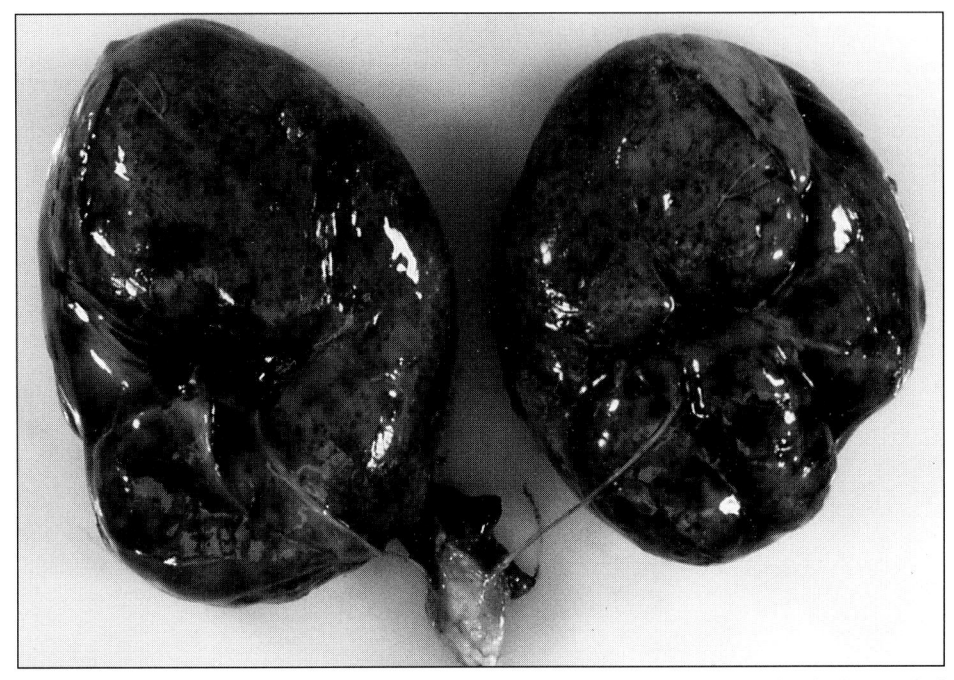

Figure 13–1. The massive kidneys have innumerable cysts represented by the dark rounded structures visible at the surface. The ureters appear threadlike and the bladder appears tiny but these structures are actually of normal size for the gestational age of the infant.

resulting in cysts of the convoluted tubules[2]; and New Zealand white rabbits, which developed cysts in the collecting ducts when given long-acting adrenal corticosteroids.[3] An accidental experimental model is found in human mothers who received indomethacin for several weeks during pregnancy. Van der Heijden et al reported six such cases in which the neonates died during the first to sixth weeks of life. Five of the six had superficial cortical cysts and ischemic damage in the deeper cortex.[4]

The issue in this case is the proper classification of renal cystic disease since the genetic information given to the family will have significant implications, not only for future pregnancies but for all the relatives.[5] The macroscopic features are characteristic for infantile or autosomal recessive polycystic kidney disease.[6] If this is indeed the diagnosis, the attendant risk of repeating in the future children of these two parents is one in four. The severe perinatal phenotype of ARPKD maps to chromosome 6p21-cen.[7] The clinical courses in affected siblings may be quite variable. Some fetuses have sonographic evidence of disease early in gestation, while siblings may not have lesions until late in the third trimester.[6] Some liveborn infants die in the first week of life, while their affected siblings can live for several months. Survival beyond the first year has recently been reported in infants who had unilateral nephrectomy, a procedure that apparently allows room for adequate diaphragmatic excursion as well as for adequate alimentation.[8]

Microscopically, the diagnosis in this case became clouded when cysts were discovered in all portions of the nephrons and collecting ducts, a feature of adult

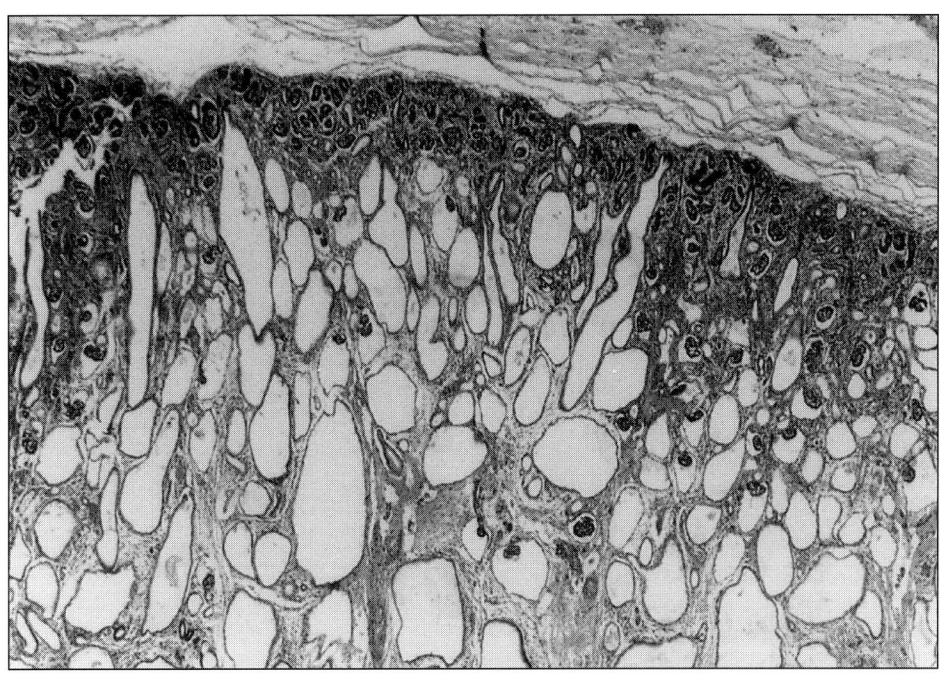

Figure 13–2. Microscopically, the cysts are fusiform in the upper cortex and tend to become rounded in the deeper renal parenchyma. This pattern is similar to that of ARPKD, but also occurs in cystic dysplastic kidneys. Features that differentiate these conditions are abundant interstitial fibrosis and formation of cysts in convoluted tubules and glomeruli, which do not occur in ARPKD.

or autosomal dominant polycystic kidney disease (ADPKD). Autosomal dominant polycystic kidney disease occurs in children and even in fetuses as early as 14 weeks' gestation.[9–13] In many reports, a parent is also affected, often subclinically. The time courses for onset and for rapidity of symptoms do not run true in these families, as had been suggested in the earlier literature.[9] Recent studies have identified genetic variants of ADPKD. The most common abnormal gene has been localized to the short arm of chromosome number 16 (16p). This condition is now designated ADPKD-1 and accounts for 80% to 90% of all cases.[14] Prenatal diagnosis has been accomplished through linkage analyses in affected families.[15] The ADPKD-2 gene is located on chromosome 4 (4q13-q23) and evidence for a third locus is indicated by finding ADPKD in families without the genes for types 1 or 2.[16] The implications for family members with ADPKD are the associated risks of hypertension and of renal failure. Cerebral vascular aneurysms are only slightly increased in affected individuals.[17]

Several features in this case are supportive of neither ARPKD nor ADPKD. The cysts involved glomeruli (Bowman's spaces), convoluted tubules, Henle's loops, and collecting ducts. These are features that exclude ARPKD. The dysplastic fibromuscular collars and immature collagenous tissue plus the reduction in normal renal parenchyma are features that exclude ADPKD. Biliary duct dysplasias and pancreatic ductal cysts are consistent with either ARPKD or ADPKD

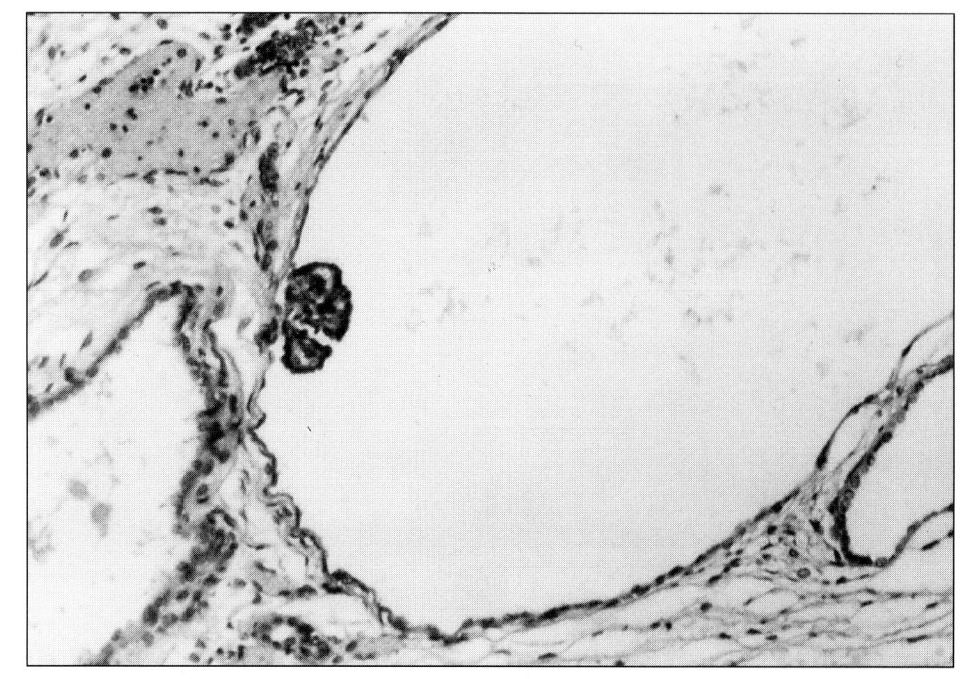

Figure 13–3. Glomerular cyst in cystic dysplastic kidney disease. This is a feature that excludes ARPKD from consideration.

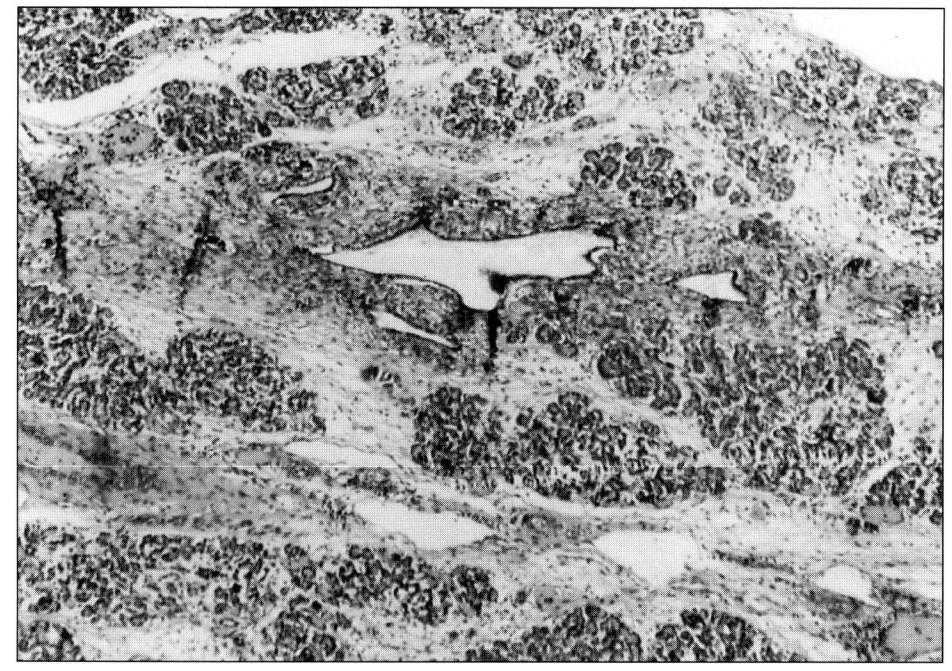

Figure 13–4. Cystic dilatation of pancreatic ducts is a feature in this case. Bile ducts in the liver were also cystic. This is a case of Ivemark's syndrome, consisting of renal cystic dysplasia, hepatic biliary dysplasia, and pancreatic ductal dysplasia.

Table 13–1. Classification of Renal Cysts[19]

Cystic renal dysplasia
Polycystic kidney disease
  Adult autosomal dominant
  Childhood autosomal recessive
Medullary cystic disease
  Sponge kidney
  Nephronophthisis—uremic
Acquired (dialysis) cystic disease
Localized simple cysts
Renal cysts in hereditary malformation syndromes
Glomerulocystic disease
Extraparenchymal renal cysts

but favor the infantile form more than the adult form.[18] A number of other conditions must be considered. The classification in Table 13–1 forms a good starting place for analyzing this case.

Cystic renal dysplasia is a condition limited to the renal parenchyma with no cystic lesions in other organs. It may be unilateral or bilateral and is often associated with obstructive uropathy. Rarely, dysplastic kidneys can have unusual features. Hsueh et al described a female born at 29 weeks' gestation who had bulging flanks, respiratory distress, and died at 36 hours of age. Both kidneys were markedly enlarged with cysts and dysplasia but they also had features of nephroblastomatosis.[20] Dysplastic kidneys may be cystic and enlarged or free of cysts and hypoplastic. When cysts are present, they can be identified in all components of the renal parenchyma. Consistent features include primitive mesenchyme and fibromuscular collars around ducts. Small islands of metaplastic cartilage may be found in the interstitial tissues.[21,22] While dysplastic kidneys occur sporadically, family members are at considerable risk for similar or related findings. Relatives have 15 times more renal dysplasia or agenesis than the general population.[23]

Renal cysts in hereditary malformation syndromes should be considered next. Jaffe[24] published a useful expanded classification of these conditions (Table 13–2).

Meckel syndrome consists of a triad of findings: occipital encephalocele, postaxial polydactyly, and cystic kidneys. Cysts may also be found in the biliary ducts and pancreatic ducts. Meckel syndrome is a lethal condition with autosomal recessive inheritance. The renal lesion is cystic dysplasia with radially oriented cysts, larger in the medullary region. Convoluted tubules and occasional Bowman's spaces are dilated. Collecting ducts are large and lined with flattened epithelial cells surrounded by thick fibromuscular collars. Glomeruli are poorly formed and nephrogenic activity is decreased in premature fetuses and infants. Interstitial connective tissue is increased and medullary zones are rudimentary, lacking vasa recta and recurrent loops. Metaplastic cartilage is usually not found, but focal extramedullary hematopoiesis is often present.[25]

The cysts in trisomy 13 are mostly glomerular, although some tubules and even ducts may have small cysts.[24] To a lesser extent and in fewer cases,

Table 13–2. Classification of Hereditary Syndromes with Cystic Kidneys[24]

ADPKD
ARPKD
Meckel
Trisomy 13
Jeune and/or Saldino-Noonan
Elejalde
Glutaric acidemia, type II
Tuberous sclerosis
von Hippel-Lindau
Ivemark

Abbreviations: ADPKD = autosomal dominant polycystic kidney disease; ARPKD = autosomal recessive polycystic kidney disease.

glomerular cysts may be found in trisomy 18 and trisomy 21. Obstructive forms of renal cystic dysplasia can be increased in trisomy 21,[26] monosomy X (Turner) syndrome,[27] and other genetically determined syndromes (see below).[28]

Several of the syndromes with osteochondrodysplasia include cystic kidneys, often with associated cysts of the biliary ducts and pancreatic ducts. Examples of these associated findings are asphyxiating thoracic dystrophy of Jeune and Saldino-Noonan and Elejalde (acrocephalopolydactylous) syndromes.[24]

Babies with glutaric acidemia, type II, have the distinction of a peculiar body odor described as resembling recently worn sweat socks. Cerebral pachygyria and facial dysmorphism are associated features along with lipid accumulation in the liver, heart, and renal tubules. Cortical cysts are present in the kidney. The medulla is devoid of cysts but has other features of dysplasia.[29]

Renal cysts occur in tuberous sclerosis and in von Hippel-Lindau disease, and renal tumors occur in both. The cysts in tuberous sclerosis are distinctive if not pathognomonic, consisting of hyperplastic pale eosinophilic cortical cysts with epithelial cells projecting into the tubular lumens, sometimes forming polypoid structures. They appear to arise from the proximal convoluted tubules. Such cysts have been identified in the kidneys of infants and are sometimes the presenting finding in patients with tuberous sclerosis.[21,30,31] Renal angiomyolipomas develop later in life. In both tuberous sclerosis and von Hippel-Lindau disease, cysts develop in the kidneys, and according to some authors, in the liver and pancreas as well.[19,32] In von Hippel-Lindau disease, a tumor suppressor gene is altered, and renal carcinomas may occur. Virtually all of the disease manifestations are limited to adults.

In some cases of the Zellweger syndrome, dysplastic cysts develop in the kidney, and hepatic fibrosis without cystic bile ducts may be an associated finding.[21]

The oral-facial-digital syndrome type 1 is a group of X-linked dominant conditions, lethal to males in utero. In girls, kidneys have thin-walled spherical cysts in the cortex that measure as much as 2 cm in diameter; the medulla contains fewer but larger cysts. All segments of the nephron and collecting ducts have cysts similar to those in adult polycystic disease.[33] Cerebro-reno-digital syn-

Table 13–3. Syndromes With Cysts of Kidney, Liver, Pancreas*

ARPKD	kidney, liver, pancreas
ADPKD	kidney, liver, pancreas
Meckel	kidney, liver, pancreas
Jeune syndrome	kidney, liver, pancreas
Zellweger	kidney, liver, pancreas
Ivemark	kidney, liver, pancreas
Saldino-Noonan	kidney, liver, pancreas
Elejalde	kidney, liver, pancreas
Trisomy 9	kidney, liver, pancreas
Trisomy 13	kidney, liver, pancreas
Glutaric acidemia, type II	kidney, liver, pancreas
Tuberous sclerosis	kidney, liver, pancreas
von Hippel-Lindau	kidney, liver, pancreas
Oro-facial-digital, type I	kidney, liver, pancreas[33]
Juvenile nephronophthisis	kidney, liver†
Majewski	kidney, liver
Carbohydrate deficient transferrin and olivopontocerebellar atrophy	kidney, liver[36]‡
Cerebro-reno-digital community	kidney[34]

Abbreviations: ADPKD = autosomal dominant polycystic kidney disease; ARPKD = autosomal recessive polycystic kidney disease.
* The syndromes without reference numbers can be found in Bernstein,[18] Cotran et al,[19] Rapola,[21] Bernstein et al,[22] Jaffe,[24] and De Girolami et al.[32]
† Fibrosis.
‡ Micronodular cirrhosis.

dromes, of which there are now at least 19, all with apparently autosomal recessive inheritance, form a community of conditions with renal cysts as one of the hallmarks.[34]

Several metabolic diseases, other than glutaric acidemia type II, show cystic changes in the kidneys. Strom et al described an autosomal recessive disorder in which the kidneys have multiple microcysts. Carbohydrate-deficient glycoprotein is a feature of this new syndrome.[35] Another condition with a carbohydrate-deficient transferrin includes renal tubular microcysts; micronodular cirrhosis of the liver; and atrophy of the cerebellum, pons, and medullary olives.[36]

In 1959, Ivemark et al[37] reported a familial syndrome consisting of dysplastic cystic kidneys with hepatic and pancreatic cysts. Since then, only a few similar cases have been added to the literature.[22,38]

Considering the previous information, the list of syndromes that have renal cysts can now be enlarged and the conditions with hepatic and pancreatic cysts are shown in Table 13–3.

Most of the previously mentioned syndromes can be ruled out on historical or morphologic grounds. After exclusion of identifiable syndromes, the diagnosis of Ivemark's renal-hepatic-pancreatic dysplasia remains[22] and that is the diagnosis rendered in this case.

DIAGNOSIS: Ivemark's renal-hepatic-pancreatic dysplasia

References

1. Crocker JFS, Brown DM, Borch RF, Vernier RL. Renal cystic disease induced in newborn rats by diphenylamine derivatives. *Am J Pathol* 1972;66:343–348.
2. Filmer RB, Carone FA, Rowland RG, Babcock JR. Adrenal corticosteroid-induced renal cystic disease in the newborn hamster. *Am J Pathol* 1973;72:461–472.
3. Perey DYE, Herdman RC, Good RA. Polycystic renal disease: A new experimental model. *Science* 1967;158:494–496.
4. van der Heijden BJ, Carlus C, Narcy F, Bavoux F, Delezoide AL, Gubler MC. Persistent anuria, neonatal death and renal microcystic lesions after prenatal exposure to indomethacin. *Am J Obstet Gynecol* 1994;171:617–623.
5. Zerres K, Völpel M-C, Weiss H. Cystic kidneys: Genetics, pathologic anatomy, clinical picture, and prenatal diagnosis. *Hum Genet* 1984;68:104–135.
6. Bronshtein M, Bar-Hava I, Blumenfeld Z. Clues and pitfalls in the early prenatal diagnosis of 'late onset' infantile polycystic kidney. *Prenat Diagn* 1992;12:293–298.
7. Guay-Woodford LM, Hopkins SD, Muecher G, Zerres K. The severe perinatal phenotype of ARPKD (autosomal recessive polycystic kidney disease) maps to chromosome 6p21-cen. *J Am Soc Nephrol* 1994;5:624.
8. Bean SA, Bednarek FJ, Primack WA. Aggressive respiratory support and unilateral nephrectomy for infants with severe perinatal autosomal recessive polycystic kidney disease. *J Pediatr* 1995;127:311–313.
9. Blyth H, Ockenden BG. Polycystic disease of kidneys and liver presenting in childhood. *J Med Genet* 1971;8:257–284.
10. Eulderink F, Hogewind BL. Renal cysts in premature children. *Arch Pathol Lab Med* 1978;102:592–595.
11. Gang DL, Herrin JT. Infantile polycystic disease of the liver and kidneys. *Clin Nephrol* 1986;25:28–36.
12. Proesmans W, Van Damme B, Casaer P, Marchal G. Autosomal dominant polycystic kidney disease in the neonatal period: Association with a cerebral arteriovenous malformation. *Pediatrics* 1982;70:971–975.
13. Waldherr R, Zerres K, Gall A, Enders H. Polycystic kidney disease in the fetus. *Lancet* 1989;2:274–275.
14. Woo D. Apoptosis and loss of renal tissue in polycystic kidney diseases. *N Engl J Med* 1995;333:18–25.
15. Turco AE, Peissel B, Rossetti S, Pignatti PF. Rapid DNA-based prenatal diagnosis of autosomal dominant polycystic kidney disease. *Arch Pediatr Adolesc Med* 1994;148:1101–1102.
16. Daoust MC, Reynolds DM, Bichet DG, Somlo S. Evidence for a third genetic locus for autosomal dominant polycystic kidney disease. *Genomics* 1995;25:733–736.
17. Chapman AB, Rubinstein D, Hughes R, et al. Intracranial aneurysms in autosomal dominant polycystic kidney disease. *N Engl J Med* 1992;327:916–920.
18. Bernstein J. Hepatic involvement in hereditary renal syndromes. *Birth Defects* 1987;23:115–130.

19. Cotran RS, Kumar V, Robbins SL. The kidney. In: Cotran RS, Kumar V, Robbins SL, eds. *Robbins Pathologic Basis of Disease.* 5th ed. Philadelphia: WB Saunders Co; 1994:935–938.
20. Hsueh C, Hsueh W, Gonzalez-Crussi F. Bilateral renal dysplasia with features of nephroblastomatosis. *Pediatr Pathol* 1987;7:437–446.
21. Rapola J. The kidneys and urinary tract. In: Wigglesworth JS, Singer DB, eds. *Textbook of Fetal and Perinatal Pathology.* Boston: Blackwell Scientific Publications, Inc; 1991:1117–1129.
22. Bernstein J, Chandra M, Creswell J, et al. Renal-hepatic-pancreatic dysplasia: A syndrome reconsidered. *Am J Med Genet* 1987;26:391–403.
23. Roodhooft AM, Birnholz JC, Holmes LB. Familial nature of congenital absence and severe dysgenesis of both kidneys. *N Engl J Med* 1984;310:1341–1345.
24. Jaffe R. The pancreas. In: Stocker JT, Dehner L, eds. *Pediatric Pathology.* Philadelphia: JB Lippincott Co; 1992:791–823.
25. Blankenberg TA, Ruebner BH, Ellis WG, Bernstein J, Dimmick JE. Pathology of renal and hepatic anomalies in Meckel syndrome. *Am J Med Genet Suppl* 1987;3:395–410.
26. Ariel I, Wells TR, Singer DB. The urinary system in Down syndrome: A study of 124 autopsy cases. *Pediatr Pathol* 1991;11(6):879–888.
27. Herman TE, Siegel MJ. Renal cysts associated with Turner's syndrome. *Pediatr Radiol* 1994;24:139–140.
28. Abt AB. Familial renal disease. *Mod Pathol* 1991;4:529–549.
29. Colevas AD, Edwards JL, Hruban RH, Mitchell GA, Valle D, Hutchins GM. Glutaric acidemia type II. *Arch Pathol Lab Med* 1988;112:1133–1139.
30. Bernstein J, Evan AP, Gardner KD Jr. Epithelial hyperplasia in human polycystic kidney diseases: Its role in pathogenesis and risk of neoplasia. *Am J Pathol* 1987;129:92–101.
31. Campos A, Figueroa ET, Gunasekaran S, Garin EH. Early presentation of tuberous sclerosis as bilateral renal cysts. *J Urol* 1993;149:1077–1079.
32. De Girolami U, Frosch MP, Anthony DC. The central nervous system. In: Cotran RS, Kumar V, Robbins SL, eds. *Robbins Pathologic Basis of Disease.* 5th ed. Philadelphia: WB Saunders Co; 1994:1335.
33. Kennedy SM, Hashida Y, Malatack JJ. Polycystic kidneys, pancreatic cysts and cystadenomatous bile ducts in the oral-facial-digital syndrome type I. *Arch Pathol Lab Med* 1991;115:519–523.
34. Lurie IW, Lazjuk GI, Korotkova IA, Cherstvoy ED. The cerebro-reno-digital syndromes: A new community. *Clin Genet* 1991;39:104–113.
35. Strom EH, Stromme P, Westvik J, Pedersen SJ. Renal cysts in the carbohydrate-deficient glycoprotein syndrome. *Pediatr Nephrol* 1993;7:253–255.
36. Chang Y, Twiss JL, Horoupian DS, Caldwell SA, Johnston KM. Inherited syndrome of infantile olivopontocerebellar atrophy, micronodular cirrhosis, and renal tubular microcysts: Review of the literature and a report of an additional case. *Acta Neuropathol* 1993;86:399–404.
37. Ivemark BI, Oldefelt P, Zetterström J. Familial dysplasia of kidneys, liver and pancreas: A probably genetically determined syndrome. *Acta Paediatr* 1959;48:1–11.
38. Strayer DS, Kissane JM. Dysplasia of the kidneys, liver and pancreas: Report of a variant of Ivemark's syndrome. *Hum Pathol* 1979;10:228–234.

Case Fourteen

Contributed by Don B. Singer, MD
Providence, Rhode Island

History

This 9-year-old girl had weight loss, chronic diarrhea, stools with occult blood, hypoalbuminemia, and anemia.

Dr Singer: The colon has multiple sessile and pedunculated juvenile polyps (JPs). Macroscopically, the polyps have smooth, bright red, glistening surfaces, sometimes with flecks of yellow-tan material. On cut section, small cystic spaces contain gray or yellow mucus or thin fluid. The stroma is edematous and inflamed. Glands are enlarged and filled with mucus. A stalk is present with the larger polyps but small polyps are sessile.

Microscopically, the stroma is infiltrated with large numbers of neutrophils and eosinophils with scattered mononuclear inflammatory elements (Figures 14–1 and 14–2). The intervening connective tissue is edematous and vessels are engorged. Granulation tissue forms beneath ulcerated surfaces (Figure 14–3). The glands are distributed haphazardly throughout the polyp and are distended with mucus. Some are rounded and large enough to be seen with the naked eye. Others are small with irregular outlines. The lining cells are typical colonic epithelial cells with varying amounts of mucus in the cytoplasm (Figure 14–4). Localized clusters of small glands are seen. Here and there, glands are lined with darker cells that are focally pseudostratified. Small papillary projections into the lumens are occasionally seen. No anaplastic features are identified in any of the polyps. Aside from these changes, one may see regenerative epithelium, especially on the surface of the polyp. Osseous metaplasia has been described in the stroma in some cases. The pathogenesis of juvenile polyps is unsettled. Some favor inflammation with retention of glandular secretions. Others favor a hamartomatous development.

Solitary juvenile polyps are the most common tumors found in the gastrointestinal tract of children. They also occur in adults as nonneoplastic lesions but on rare occasion are associated with adenomatous or carcinomatous changes in the gastrointestinal tract.[1] The juvenile polyposis syndromes are associated with multiple nonadenomatous and nonhamartomatous polyps, usually isolated in the colon but sometimes involving the small intestine or stomach. These must be differentiated from other multiple polyposis syndromes since some of the latter commonly lead to carcinoma of the colon (Table 14–1).[2]

Gardner syndrome has an autosomal dominant pattern of inheritance with adenomatous polyps of the colon and tumors of the skull or mandible, skin, and soft tissue. In Turcot's syndrome, a condition with autosomal recessive inheri-

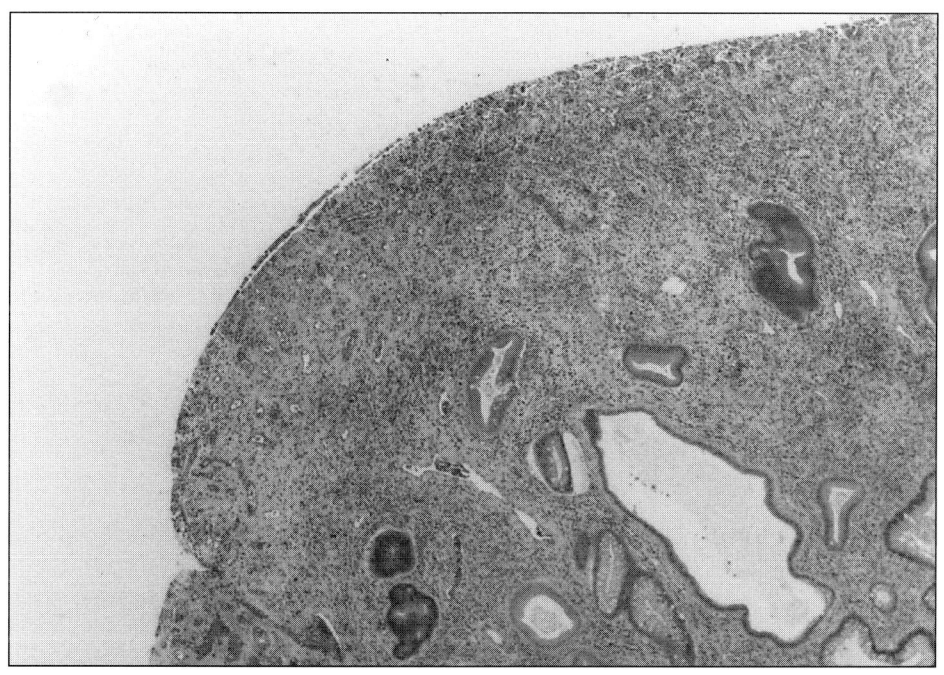

Figure 14-1. Edge of juvenile polyp with eroded surface. The stroma is filled with inflammatory cells and the glands are separated by the inflamed stroma.

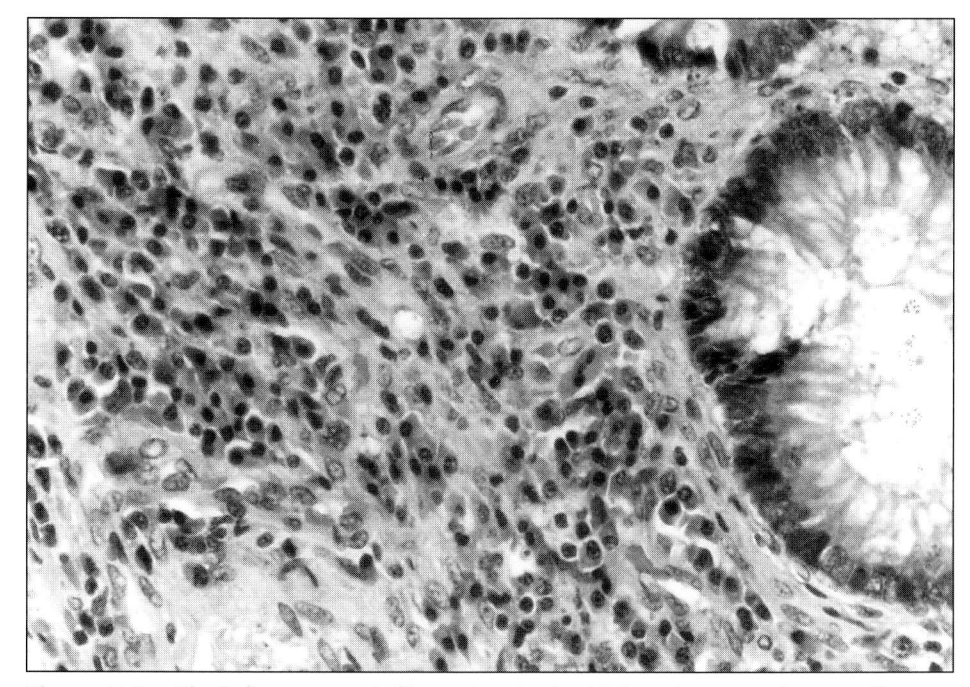

Figure 14-2. The inflammatory infiltrate is mixed with lymphocytes, plasma cells, neutrophils, and eosinophils.

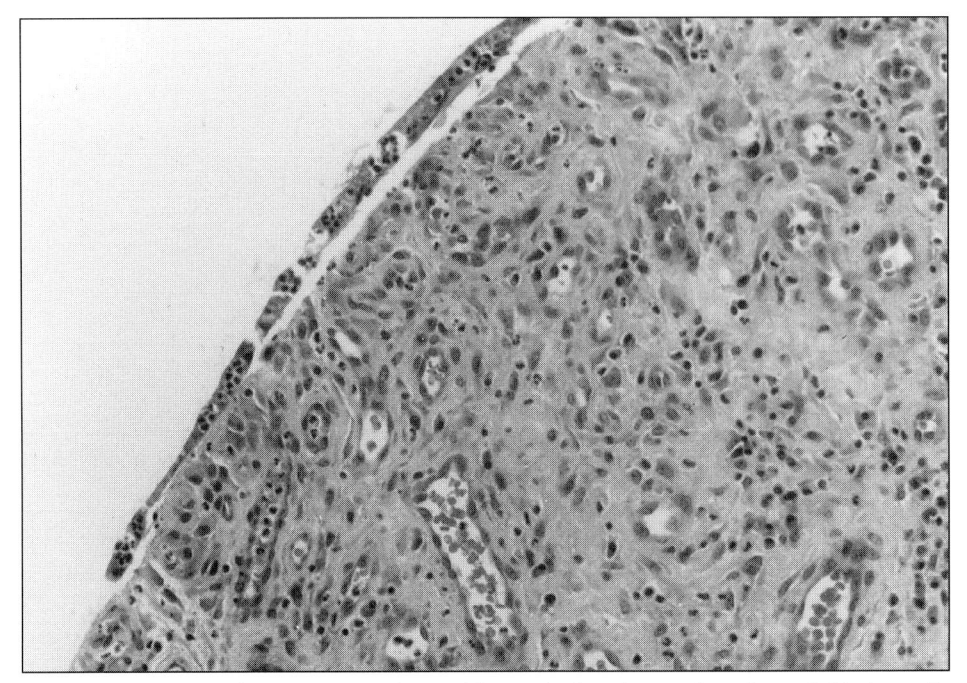

Figure 14-3. Granulation tissue is formed beneath the ulcerated surface of this juvenile polyp.

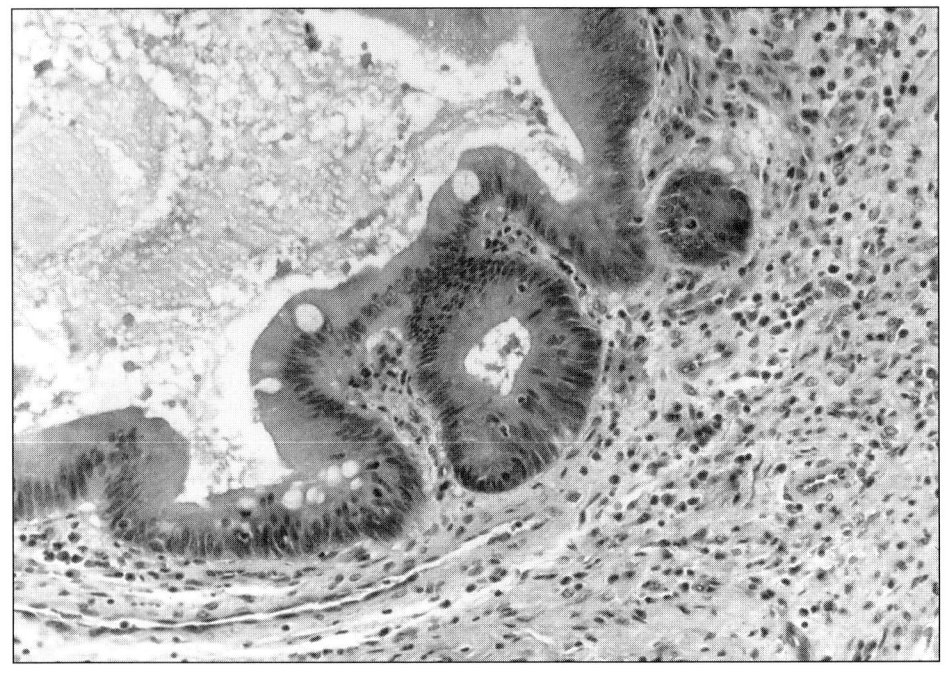

Figure 14-4. Glands are lined by benign colonic epithelium with varying amounts of mucus.

Table 14–1. Classification of GI Polyps in Children*

Adenomatous	Inflammatory	Hamartomatous
Isolated polyp	Isolated polyp	Peutz-Jeghers
Gardner syndrome	Juvenile polyposis coli	Cowden disease
Turcot syndrome	Generalized juvenile polyposis	
Familial adenomatous polyps		

*Modified, with permission from Winter.[2]

tance, familial adenomatous polyposis is associated with glioma or medulloblastoma.[3,4] Hamilton et al have recently identified the gene for familial adenomatous polyposis coli in 10 families with Turcot's syndrome. Medulloblastomas occurred in these families with a frequency 92 times that in the general population.[5] Familial adenomatous polyposis has also been reported together with hepatoblastomas.[6,7] The genetic defect for familial polyposis coli is a deletion on the long arm of chromosome 5. Phillips et al found nine cases of hepatoblastoma in patients with familial adenomatous polyps and the characteristic 5q deletion.[8] These authors estimated that this association would occur by chance once every 500 years.

Peutz-Jeghers syndrome consists of hamartomatous polyps in the small intestine, and sometimes in the colon or stomach, all usually with low malignant potential. Punctate pigmentation of the lips and buccal mucosa is present in early life. Peutz-Jeghers syndrome has an autosomal dominant inheritance pattern.[4] Malignant tumors of the lung, breast, and pancreas are reported in adults. These patients are also prone to develop gonadal sex cord stromal tumors, which are usually benign.[9] Cowden syndrome has multiple hamartomas of ectodermal, endodermal, and mesodermal derivation, with a high incidence of malignant tumors of the breast and thyroid gland. Skin lesions are common, especially tricholemmomas. Hamartomatous polyps develop in the gastrointestinal tract. The pattern of inheritance is autosomal dominant. Williard et al analyzed *ras* oncogene, HER-2/*neu* oncogene, and pS-2, the estrogen inducible gene. These oncogenes are commonly associated with breast cancers, but none were amplified in their patient with Cowden syndrome.[10]

Juvenile polyposis syndromes usually occur in the first decade, as in this case.[1] An exception is the Cronkhite-Canada syndrome, which consists of multiple juvenile colonic polyps, alopecia, nail atrophy, and hyperpigmentation of the skin. This syndrome is nonfamilial, and usually occurs in older adults.[11,12]

Juvenile polyposis coli (JPC) is limited to the colon while in generalized juvenile polyposis (GJP), polyps are distributed in the colon, small bowel, and stomach.[13] The distinction may be arbitrary, and these two conditions may actually represent a continuum.[4]

Clinically, hematochezia is the most common sign of JPC. Failure to thrive and rectal prolapse have been reported. Malignancy is not a clinically significant problem, although occasional cases have been reported years following the initial diagnosis. During childhood, polyps in JPC may be treated conservatively, ie, with removal of polyps at repeated colonoscopic examinations.[14] This is the course followed in our patient who, at age 11 years, has had approximately 200 polyps removed from her colon, some of which have had minimal adenomatous changes. She seems to be thriving but new polyps are recognized at each colonoscopic examination.

With GJP, patients may have malabsorption, hemorrhage, intussusception, hypoalbuminemia, diarrhea, clubbing, etc, due to the extracolonic involvement. In GJP adenocarcinomas and adenomatous changes are important considerations. Neoplasia can develop in the stomach, small intestine, or colon, and surveillance of the gastrointestinal tract throughout life is necessary.[2] Predicting which cases will develop carcinoma and which ones won't is difficult.[15] In one family, 21 members had polyps and/or carcinoma in the colon, stomach, or both. Polyps only were found in 10, carcinoma only in 6, and both polyps and carcinoma in 5.[16] Among 57 patients with one or more juvenile polyps, 10 (18%) developed colorectal neoplasia. Six of these had adenomatous epithelium in one or more juvenile polyps and one had frank carcinoma in a juvenile polyp. Nine of the 10 with carcinoma had at least three juvenile polyps, and eight of the nine had a family history of juvenile polyps. The carcinomas developed in young adults (mean age 37 years).[17]

Examining every part of every specimen microscopically is important. Heiss et al[18] reported three children, ages 3, 11, and 11 years, each of whom had multiple colonic polyps. Adenomatous polyps were scattered in a field of juvenile polyps, and atypia occurred in some of the polyps in two cases. In the case reported by Atsumi et al,[19] a young adult male had 23 juvenile polyps removed during colonoscopy. None of the polyps had adenomatous changes. Ten months later, the resected rectosigmoid colon had multiple polyps with adenomatous changes. In another report, a mother 40 years of age and her son, 7 years of age, each underwent a colectomy. Both colons contained predominantly juvenile polyps. The mother's specimen had numerous tubular adenomas and one severely dysplastic villous adenoma, 5 cm in diameter, without invasion. The son's specimen had adenomatous change in several juvenile polyps.[20] In still another kindred, some of the patients had polyps with villous adenomatous changes, at least one of which was associated with cancer in the same polyp.[15] Lipper et al reported a similar example of villous adenoma in a patient with multiple juvenile polyps but without carcinomatous change.[21] These specimens suggest a sequence of change from juvenile polyps to adenomatous polyps to villous adenomas and to cancer.

It is evident that an accurate classification is needed.

DIAGNOSIS: Juvenile polyposis coli

References

1. Ming S-C. Epithelial polyps of the stomach. In: Goldman H, Ming S-C, eds. *Pathology of the Gastrointestinal Tract*. Philadelphia: WB Saunders Co; 1992: 563–564.

2. Winter H. Intestinal polyps. In: Durie PR, Walker WA, Hamilton JR, Walker-Smith JA, Watkins JB, eds. *Pediatric Gastrointestinal Disease: Pathophysiology, Diagnosis, Management.* Philadelphia: BC Decker Inc; 1991: 739–753.
3. Kropilak M, Fazio VW, Lavery IL, McGannon E. Brain tumors in familial adenomatous polyposis. *Dis Colon Rectum* 1989;32:778–782.
4. Dahms BB. The gastrointestinal tract. In: Stocker JT, Dehner LP, ed. *Pediatric Pathology.* Philadelphia: JB Lippincott Co; 1992:690–692.
5. Hamilton SR, Liu B, Parsons RE, et al. The molecular basis of Turcot's syndrome. *N Engl J Med* 1995;332:839–847.
6. Giardello FM, Offerhaus JA, Krush AJ, et al. Risk of hepatoblastoma in familial adenomatous polyposis. *J Pediatr* 1991;119:766–768.
7. Hartley AL, Birch JM, Kelsey AM, Morris Jones PHM, Harris M, Blair V. Epidemiological and familial aspects of hepatoblastoma. *Med Pediatr Oncol* 1990;18:103–109.
8. Phillips M, Dicks-Mireaux C, Kingston J, et al. Hepatoblastoma and polyposis coli (familial adenomatous polyposis). *Med Pediatr Oncol* 1989;17:441–447.
9. Spigelman AD, Murday V, Phillips RK. Cancer and the Peutz-Jeghers syndrome. *Gut* 1989;30:1588–1590.
10. Williard W, Borden P, Bol R, Tiwari R, Osborne M. Cowden's disease: A case report with analyses at the molecular level. *Cancer* 1992;69:2969–2974.
11. Cronkhite LW Jr., Canada WJ. Generalized gastrointestinal polyposis. *N Engl J Med* 1955;252:1011–1015.
12. Daniel ES, Ludwig SL, Lewin KJ, et al. The Cronkhite-Canada syndrome: An analysis of clinical and pathologic features and therapy in 55 patients. *Medicine* 1982;61:293–309.
13. Sachatello CR, Pickren JW, Grance JT Jr. Generalized juvenile gastrointestinal polyposis. *Gastroenterology* 1970;58:699–708.
14. Sturniolo GC, Montino MC, Dall'Igna F, et al. Familial juvenile polyposis coli: results of endoscopic treatment and surveillance in two sisters. *Gastrointest Endoscopy* 1993;39:561–565.
15. Subramony C, Scott-Conner CEH, Skelton D, Hall TJ. Familial juvenile polyposis: Study of a kindred—Evolution of polyps and relationship to gastrointestinal carcinoma. *Am J Clin Pathol* 1994;102:91–97.
16. Stemper TJ, Kent TH, Summers RW. Juvenile polyposis and gastrointestinal carcinoma: A study of a kindred. *Ann Intern Med* 1975;83:639–646.
17. Giardello FM, Hamilton SR, Kern SE, et al. Colorectal neoplasia in juvenile polyposis or juvenile polyps. *Arch Dis Child* 1991;66:971–975.
18. Heiss KF, Schaffner D, Ricketts RR, Winn K. Malignant risk in juvenile polyposis coli: Increasing documentation in the pediatric age group. *J Pediatr Surg* 1993;28:1188–1193.
19. Atsumi M, Kawamoto K, Ebisui S, et al. A case report of juvenile polyposis with adenomatous change and a review of 34 cases reported in Japan. *Gastroenterol Jpn* 1991;26:523–529.
20. O'Riordan DS, O'Dwyer PJ, Cullen AF, McDermott EW, Murphy JJ. Familial juvenile polyposis coli and colorectal cancer. *Cancer* 1991;68:889–892.
21. Lipper S, Kahn LB, Sandler RS, Varma V. Multiple juvenile polyposis: A study of the pathogenesis of juvenile polyps and their relationship to colonic adenomas. *Hum Pathol* 1981;12:804–813.

Case Fifteen

Contributed by Aleli Siongco, MD
Fresno, California

History

The patient is a 13-year-old girl with a normal menstrual history who presented with abdominal enlargement and pain. Admitting workup showed the presence of ascites, hypoalbuminemia, and a possible ovarian mass. The radiologic examination showed a right adnexal mass with possible partial torsion. At laparotomy, a right salpingo-oophorectomy was performed. The patient remains well after 1 year.

Dr Dehner: The right ovary weighed 135 g and measured 11 cm in greatest dimension. On the cut surface, the capsule has a thickened and fibrotic appearance. The surface has a solid tan mucoid appearance with focal yellowish, firm areas (Figure 15–1). Several histologic patterns are apparent in different areas of the tumor. The thickened cortex and subcortical region are separated from the more solidly cellular, lobular, and pseudolobular areas by a hypocellular myxomatous zone (Figure 15–2). Some of the latter areas are also accompanied by collagen deposition, producing a fibromyxomatous stroma (Figure 15–3, top and bottom). The lobular or pseudolobular foci are moderately cellular and are accompanied by a prominent network of thin-walled vascular spaces. Small cords and nests of polygonal cells, individual polygonal cells, and a background of loosely arrayed delicate spindle cells are the cellular elements of the pseudolobules (Figure 15–4). The polygonal cells have clear to slightly granular eosinophilic cytoplasm. Occasional polygonal cells have a signet ring–like appearance with the curvilinear displacement of the nucleus by a clear vacuole (see Figure 15–4, arrow). The nuclei of the polygonal cells have delicate, evenly dispersed chromatin. Mitotic figures are inapparent. A mucicarmine stain failed to demonstrate the presence of cytoplasmic mucin.

The differential diagnosis of this unilateral solid ovarian neoplasm includes massive edema of the ovary, myxoma, hemangioma, fibromatosis, Kruckenberg tumor, and sclerosing stromal tumor. Since Kruckenberg tumors are bilateral by definition, this diagnosis can be dismissed from further consideration on the basis of clinical findings and the absence of mucin in the few signet ring–like cells. Kruckenberg tumors generally present in older patients, but they are known to occur in women late in the second or third decade of life.[1,2] A poorly differentiated adenocarcinoma of the stomach is the most common primary site.

With the exception of the hemangioma, which rarely occurs in the ovary, the other entities in the differential diagnosis have several overlapping pathologic features. For instance, there are areas within this tumor that are similar to those seen in MOE, myxoma, and fibromatosis, but it is the lobular or pseudolobular

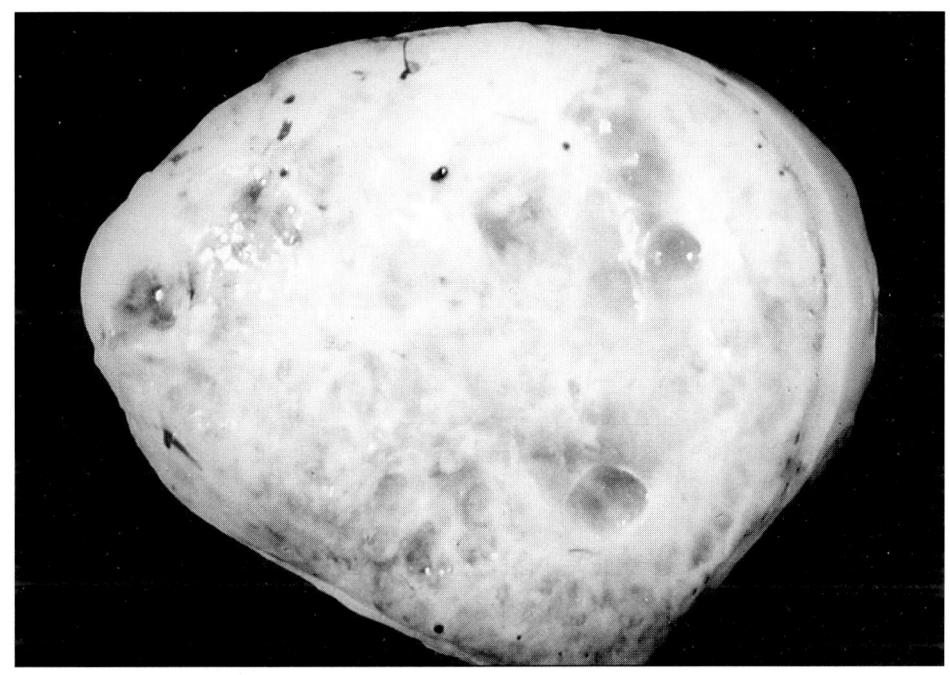

Figure 15–1. The right ovary has a thickened cortex and a discrete solid mass with focal cysts. An irregular trabecular and lobular surface is seen on cross section.

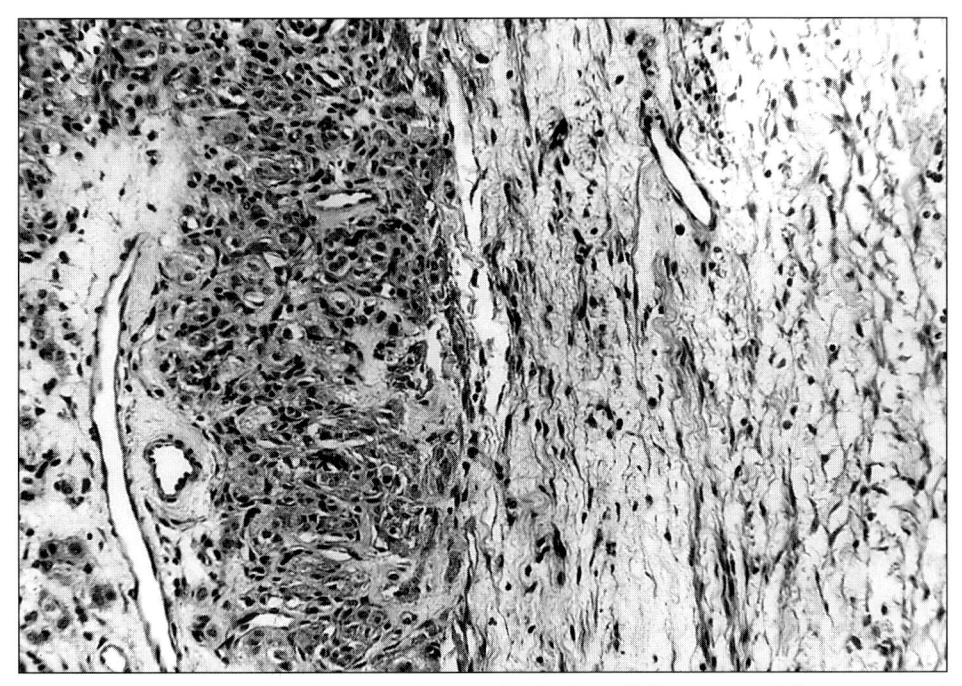

Figure 15–2. The interface between the pseudolobular cellular areas and the compressed fibrous cortex is composed of loose myxomatous tissue.

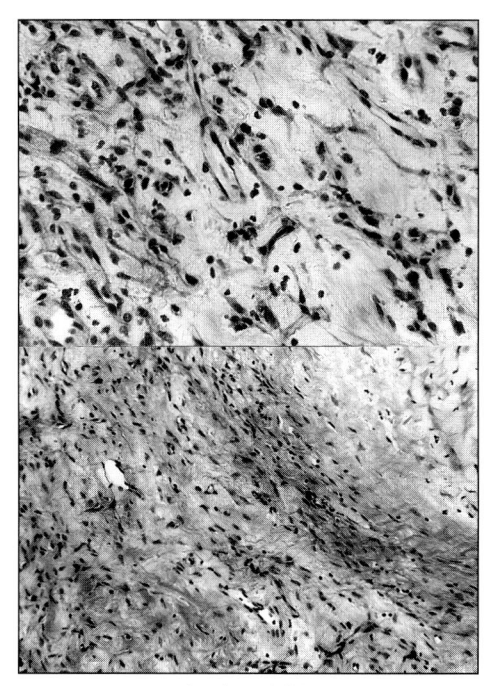

Figure 15–3. Extensive myxomatous (top) and fibromatous (bottom) areas of the sclerosing stromal tumor are also features of massive ovarian edema, myxoma, and fibromatosis.

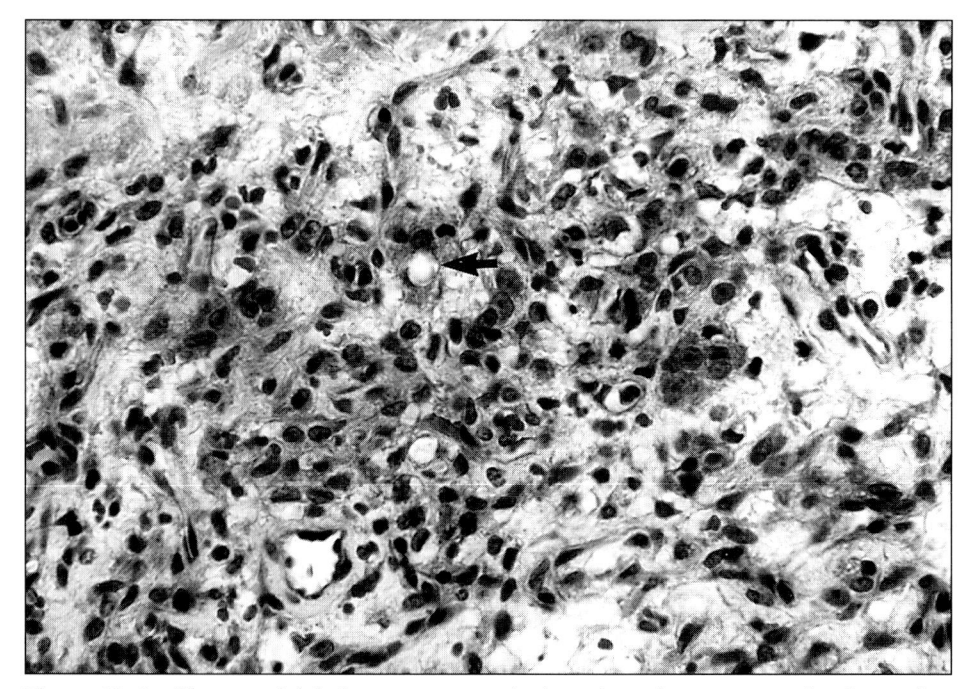

Figure 15–4. The pseudolobules are composed of condensed aggregates of polygonal to spindle-shaped cells with clear to pale eosinophilic cytoplasm. Occasional signet ring–like cells may be identified (arrow).

areas that are the characteristic microscopic features of sclerosing stromal tumor of the ovary.

Primary ovarian neoplasms in the first two decades of life are uncommon when compared to their relative frequency later in life. The distribution of tumor subtypes varies substantially between adults and children.[3] Whereas two-thirds of benign and malignant ovarian neoplasms in adults are one or another type of common surface or müllerian-epithelial–derived tumors, almost the same proportion of primary ovarian neoplasms in children are germ cell–teratomatous tumors. Only 15% to 20% of ovarian neoplasms in children are derived from the common surface epithelium. Sex cord–stromal neoplasms are equally uncommon in children and adults, comprising 10% to 15% of cases.

Under the general category of granulosa-stromal cell tumors, there are two major subcategories, granulosa cell tumor and thecoma-fibroma.[3] The sclerosing stromal tumor is included as one of the several distinctive tumor types in the subcategory of thecoma-fibroma. The fibroma and thecoma comprise more than 90% of all neoplasms in the subcategory of thecoma-fibroma and for that matter, the general category of granulosa-stromal cell tumors as well.

The sclerosing stromal tumor (SST) is one of the uncommon neoplasms of the ovary.[3,4] In a literature review through 1989, approximately 80 cases had been reported since 1973.[5] This is a tumor with a predilection for younger women, typically under the age of 30 years in 80% or more of cases. In the original series, Chalvardjian and Scully[6] reported 10 patients between the ages of 14 and 51 years, six of whom were 25 years old or less. Irregular menstrual bleeding was the most common clinical presentation. Overt dyshormonal manifestations were not apparent in any women in the initial series, but there is at least one case of a 29-year-old pregnant female who developed masculinizing signs.[7] These tumors are unilateral, without exception to date, and may be quite large in some instances, weighing in excess of 600 g. A compressed rim of ovarian stroma is typically present around a fibromyxomatous mass with variable microscopic features. The cellular constituents are represented by polygonal and spindle cells. The vacuolated character of the polygonal cells may cause concern about the possibility of signet-ring cells and a Kruckenberg tumor. The histogenesis of the SST is still unresolved, but the tumor cells are immunoreactive for vimentin and muscle-specific actin.[4,8] Electron microscopy and immunohistochemistry have suggested a possible smooth muscle derivation for this tumor. There has also been speculation in the literature about the possible relationship between the SST and myxoma, massive ovarian edema, and fibromatosis of the ovary.[9,10] It should not be a surprise that the thecoma and SST share several common morphologic features.[9] Whereas the thecoma and fibroma tend to be histologically uniform neoplasms, the SST has a variable morphosis both grossly and microscopically.

The SST is a type of sex cord–stromal tumor in the subcategory of "tumors in the thecoma-fibroma group," which includes the thecoma (typical and luteinized), fibroma-fibrosarcoma, stromal tumor with minor sex cord elements, and signet-ring cell stromal tumor.[3,4]

DIAGNOSIS: Sclerosing stromal tumor of the ovary

References

1. Yakushiji M, Tazaki T, Nishimura H, Kato T. Kruckenberg tumors of the ovary: A clinicopathologic analysis of 112 cases. *Acta Obstet Gynecol Jpn* 1987;39:479–485.
2. Gargano G, Catino A, Correale M, et al. Kruckenberg tumor: A report of six cases. *Eur J Gynecol Oncol* 1992;13:431–435.
3. Young RH, Clement PB, Scully RE. The ovary. In: Sternberg SS, ed. *Diagnostic Surgical Pathology*. 2nd ed. New York: Raven Press; 1994:2195–2279.
4. Young RH, Scully RE. Sex-cord stromal, steroid cell, and other ovarian tumors with endocrine and paraneoplastic manifestations. In: *Blaustein's Pathology of the Female Genital Tract*. 4th ed. New York: Springer-Verlag; 1994:783–847.
5. Saitoh A, Tsutsumi Y, Osamura RY, Watanabe K. Sclerosing stromal tumor of the ovary: Immunohistochemical and electron microscopic demonstration of smooth-muscle differentiation. *Arch Pathol Lab Med* 1989;113:372–376.
6. Chalvardjian A, Scully RE. Sclerosing stromal tumors of the ovary. *Cancer* 1973;31:664–670.
7. Cashell AW, Cohen ML. Masculinizing sclerosing stromal tumor of the ovary during pregnancy. *Gynecol Oncol* 1991;43:281–285.
8. Shaw JA, Dabbs DJ, Geisinger KR. Sclerosing stromal tumor of the ovary: An ultrastructural and immunohistochemical analysis with histogenetic considerations. *Ultrastruct Pathol* 1992;16:363–377.
9. Costa MJ, Morris R, DeRose PB, Cohen C. Histologic and immunohistochemical evidence for considering ovarian myxoma as a variant of the thecoma-fibroma group of ovarian stromal tumors. *Arch Pathol Lab Med* 1993;117:802–808.
10. Costa MJ, Thomas W, Majmudar B, Hewan-Lowe K. Ovarian myxoma: Ultrastructural and immunohistochemical findings. *Ultrastruct Pathol* 1992;16:429–438.

Case Sixteen

Contributed by Stephen H. Kassel, MD
Fresno, California

History

The patient is a 7-year-old girl with precocious pseudopuberty who was found to have a right ovarian mass. A multicystic mass occupied the right ovary and was excised. The patient remains well 1 year after surgery.

Dr Dehner: The right ovary measures 8 cm in greatest dimension and weighs 160 g. Its external surface is smooth and has a tan-pink color. On sectioning, the mass has a multicystic appearance with cysts measuring up to 1.2 cm in diameter (Figure 16–1). The cysts are filled with a dark yellow, thick fluid and have smooth inner surfaces without any irregularities. Microscopically, the cysts are lined by small, relatively uniform cells with either a regular stratified appearance or structures with microfollicular or Call-Exner body–like features (Figure 16–2, top and bottom). The Call-Exner bodies have also grown into the supporting stroma of the septa; delicate compressed cords of tumor cells in seeming transition from the lining granulosa cells are present in the septa (Figure 16–3, top and bottom). The nuclei are angulated and many have nuclear grooves.

The differential diagnosis of this multicystic mass is limited to a granulosa cell tumor vs. multiple follicular cysts in an otherwise normal ovary; however, there was no identifiable residual ovarian parenchyma other than the residual cortex. Most follicular cysts have a layer of luteinized cells beneath the granulosa cells, but luteinized cells are not present in this case. The presence of Call-Exner bodies throughout this multicystic ovary is not an expected finding in a multicystic or sclerocystic ovary with follicular cysts.

The previous case (Case 15) was also an example of a sex cord–stromal neoplasm in the broad category of granulosa-stromal cell tumors but in the subcategory of thecoma-fibroma. This case is a representative tumor type in the same broad category of granulosa-stromal cell tumors, but rather than in the subcategory of thecoma-fibroma, it is an example of a granulosa cell tumor (GCT). There are two basic subtypes of GCT: adult and juvenile.[1] Among the sex cord–stromal neoplasms of the ovary in children, 50% or greater of all cases are juvenile GCTs. Precocious puberty is the most common clinical presentation of the juvenile GCT. However, the present case is a rare example of an adult GCT presenting in a similar manner to a juvenile GCT. A virtually identical case to this one has been reported by Arisaka et al in a 6-year-old girl.[2] As further documentation of its functional character, our patient had a preoperative estradiol level of 7.8 ng/dL (normal: less than 1.5 ng/dL).

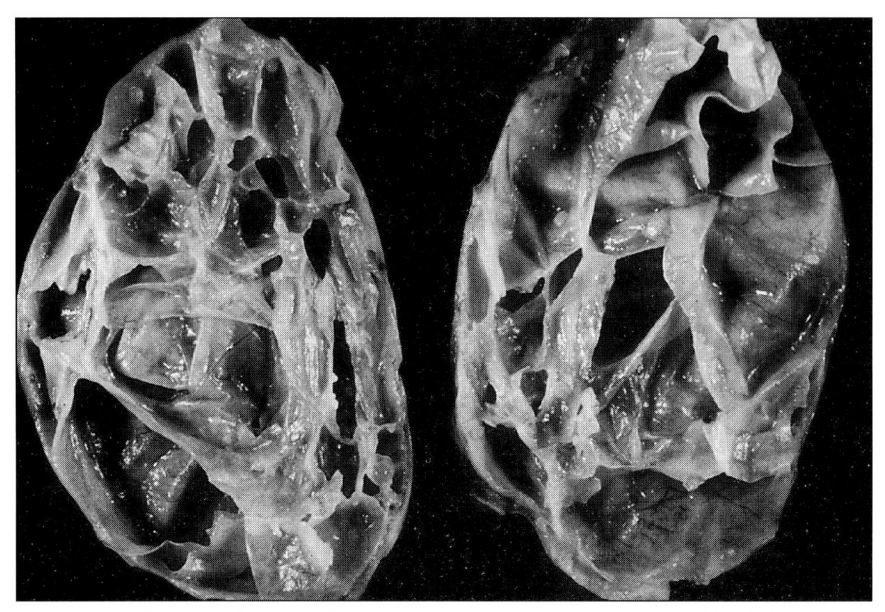

104 *Placental, Neonatal, and Pediatric Pathology*

Figure 16–1. The ovary has a multicystic appearance on cut surface. All of the cysts have smooth, glistening surfaces.

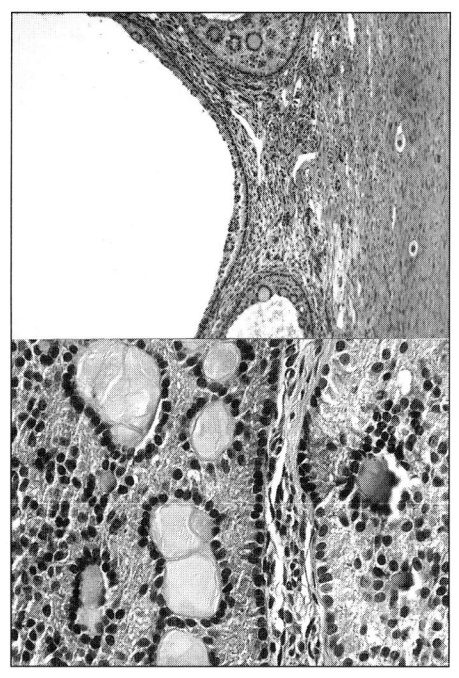

Figure 16–2. There is an intact cortex, but the remainder of the ovary has been replaced by multiple cysts in which the lining epithelium is composed of granulosa cells arranged as Call-Exner bodies (top). The characteristic Call-Exner bodies are microfollicles with central eosinophilic material (bottom).

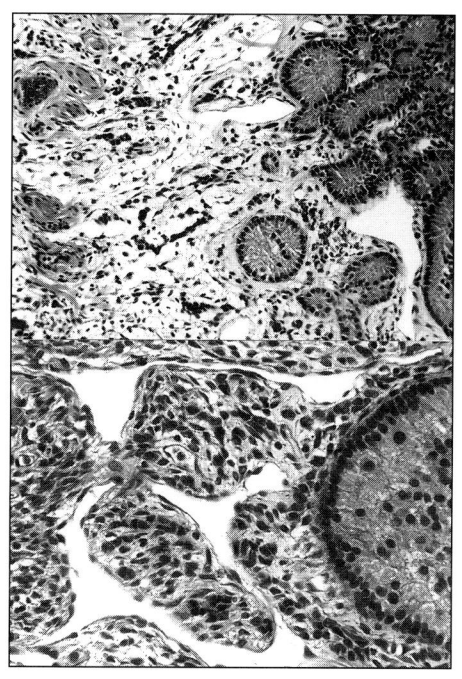

Figure 16–3. The Call-Exner bodies invade into the underlying stroma (top). In the septal areas, the tumor cells are also arranged into narrow strands or nodules of stromal cells with the same cytologic features as granulosa cells in the Call-Exner bodies (bottom).

The adult GCT has several morphologic patterns including the solid and cystic (unicystic or multicystic) and has the following microscopic patterns: solid, microfollicular, macrofollicular, insular, trabecular, gyriform, and solid-tubular.[1] In our case, we have an example of the macrofollicular variant of adult GCT, which in adults has been associated with masculinizing signs.

It is estimated that 1% or fewer adult GCTs present before puberty.[1] In fact, the overwhelming majority of adult GCTs are diagnosed in women over the age of 40 years with a peak age between 50 and 55 years. In contrast, the juvenile GCT as a rule is diagnosed before 30 years of age, as shown by Young et al, who reported an average age of 13 years, and 44% of patients were 10 years old or less at diagnosis.[3] A juvenile GCT may present in the neonatal period. Over 80% of prepubertal patients present with precocious puberty. The juvenile GCT, like the adult variant, is unilateral in greater than 95% of cases and is grossly either solid and cystic or exclusively solid in 85% of cases (Figure 16–4).[3-5] A purely cystic juvenile GCT is found in only 10% to 15% of cases. There are two basic histologic patterns of juvenile GCT, diffuse and follicular. The follicles tend to vary in size, have a luteinized appearance, and lack the nuclear grooves of the adult GCT (Figure 16–5). The solid areas are composed of cells with thecomatous features. Mitotic figures may be abundant, and nuclear atypism and anaplasia may be disturbing in their degree. Malignant behavior with multiple recurrences and aggressive intra-abdominal growth occurs in 5% to 7% of cases.[3] Since most juvenile GCTs are pathologic stage I, most patients do well following unilateral salpingo-oophorectomy.

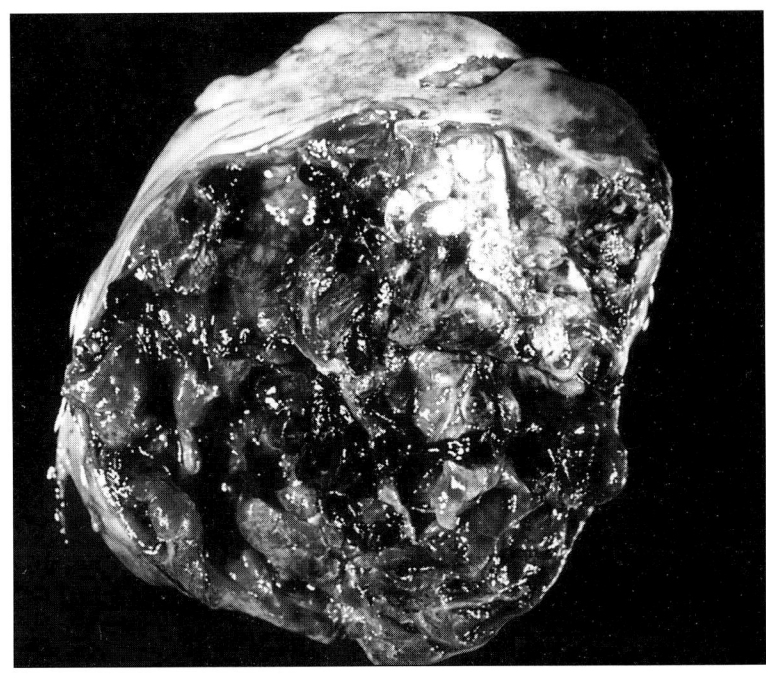

Figure 16–4. Juvenile granulosa cell tumor has its usual gross appearance as a solid and cystic mass with extensive areas of hemorrhage.

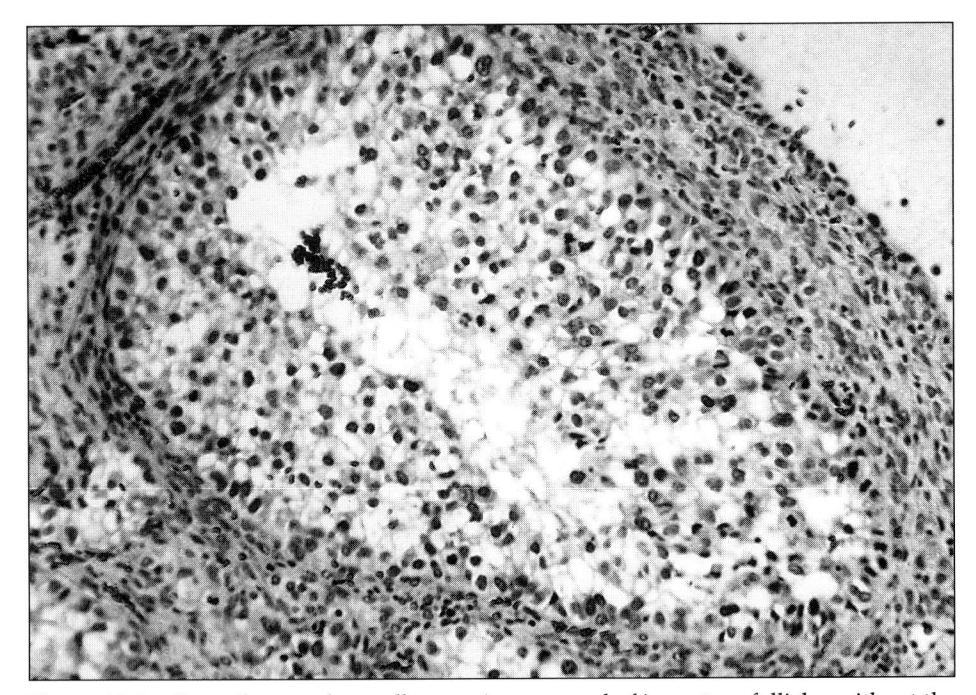

Figure 16–5. Juvenile granulosa cell tumor is composed of immature follicles without the formation of Call-Exner bodies. Mucoid basophilic secretions are present in the center of the follicles.

Our patient presented with precocious puberty, which is seen in a girl who shows signs of sexual development before 8 years of age and in a boy before 9 years of age. Precocious puberty is divided into three types: central, peripheral, and peripheral with central activation.[6] The National Institute of Health's series included 129 children with precocious puberty; there was a female predilection (74% of cases), the most common category was idiopathic central precocious puberty (48% of cases), and 60 of 62 patients were female. Our patient with a functional neoplasm of the ovary is an example of peripheral precocious puberty. Other peripheral causes include ovarian cysts, congenital adrenal hyperplasia, and adrenal cortical neoplasms.[7-9]

DIAGNOSIS: Adult type granulosa cell tumor, macrofollicular variant

References

1. Young RH, Scully RE. Sex cord-stromal, steroid cell, and other ovarian tumors with endocrine, paraendocrine, and paraneoplastic manifestation. In: Kurman RJ, ed. *Blaustein's Pathology of the Female Genital Tract*. 4th ed. New York: Springer-Verlag; 1994:783–847.
2. Arisaka O, Matsumoto T, Hosaka A, et al. Cystic adult granulosa cell tumor causing precocious pseudopuberty in a six-year-old girl. *Acta Pediatr* 1992;81:1061–1064.
3. Young RH, Dickesin GR, Scully RE. Juvenile granulosa cell tumors of the ovary: A clinicopathologic analysis of 125 cases. *Am J Surg Pathol* 1984;8:575–596.
4. Ayhan A, Tuncer ZS, Tuncer R, et al. Granulosa cell tumor of the ovary: A clinicopathologic evaluation of 60 cases. *Eur J Gynaecol Oncol* 1994;15:320–324.
5. Piura B, Nemet D, Yanai-Inbar I, et al. Granulosa cell tumor of the ovary: A study of 18 cases. *J Surg Oncol* 1994;55:71–77.
6. Pescovitz OH, Comite F, Heuch K, et al. The NIH experience with precocious puberty: Diagnostic subgroups and response to short-term luteinizing hormone releasing hormone analogue therapy. *J Pediatr* 1986;108:47–54.
7. Sinnecker G, Willig RP, Stahrake N, Braendle W. Precocious pseudopuberty associated with multiple ovarian follicular cysts and low plasma oestradiol concentrations. *Eur J Pediatr* 1989;148:600–602.
8. Arisaka O, Shimora N, Nakayama Y, et al. Ovarian cysts in precocious puberty. *Clin Pediatr* 1989;28:44–47.
9. Millar DM, Blake JM, Stringer DA, et al. Prepubertal ovarian cyst formation: 5 years' experience. *Obstet Gynecol* 1993;81:434–438.

Case Seventeen

Contributed by Don B. Singer, MD
Providence, Rhode Island

History

This 6-year-old boy had a history of neuromuscular disease and a chronic seizure disorder from early infancy. His nephew also has failure to thrive and hypotonicity. Persistent and progressive hypotension developed and eventually required epinephrine to sustain his blood pressure and pulse, but dysrhythmias supervened and he died.

Dr Singer: The sections are of spinal cord and show subtle vacuolization in the posterior columns (Figure 17–1) and, in the thoracic segments, neuronal degeneration in Clark's nucleus. With Luxol fast blue stains, the demyelination is obvious (Figure 17–2). Cardiac lesions consist of myocardial fibrosis and a dilated, hypertrophic left ventricle (Figure 17–3). Muscle atrophy and fatty infiltration are severe. These and other findings in the autopsy are characteristic of Friedreich's ataxia (FA).

FA usually begins in early childhood. Symptoms may rarely develop in infancy or may be delayed until after the third decade.[1] Older onset is associated with fewer skeletal deformities but the neurophysiologic findings, results of sural nerve biopsy, and radiologic findings are similar to those of typical early onset disease.[2] The most prominent sign is ataxia; also common are nystagmus, weakness, spasticity, kyphoscoliosis, pes cavus, and progressive cardiomyopathy.[3] Deep sensation is impaired (vibration, position, and joint sense), and deep tendon reflexes are usually absent. Variants of FA may have preserved deep tendon reflexes.[4] Gait abnormality is first noticed by parents. Dysarthria appears more slowly and becomes consistent after 5 to 10 years. The plantar response is positive in almost 90% of cases in the early stages of disease. Clubfeet are characteristic skeletal deformities.[1]

Three neuronal systems degenerate in FA. First, cells are lost in the dorsal root ganglia, producing axonal degeneration and demyelination in the fasciculus gracilis and peripheral nerves and accounting for ataxia. Second, motor neurons in the cortex develop axonal degeneration with corticospinal tract demyelination, producing weakness and spasticity. Third, loss of neurons in Clarke's column causes axonal degeneration and demyelination, contributing to ataxia. Progression is associated with dysphagia, inanition, and congestive heart failure.[3] Death occurs within 10 to 20 years but survival for more than 50 years following onset of symptoms is possible.[5]

In FA, the neuropathologic lesions are most obvious in the spinal cord, where atrophy of the posterior columns is evident even on macroscopic inspection. The

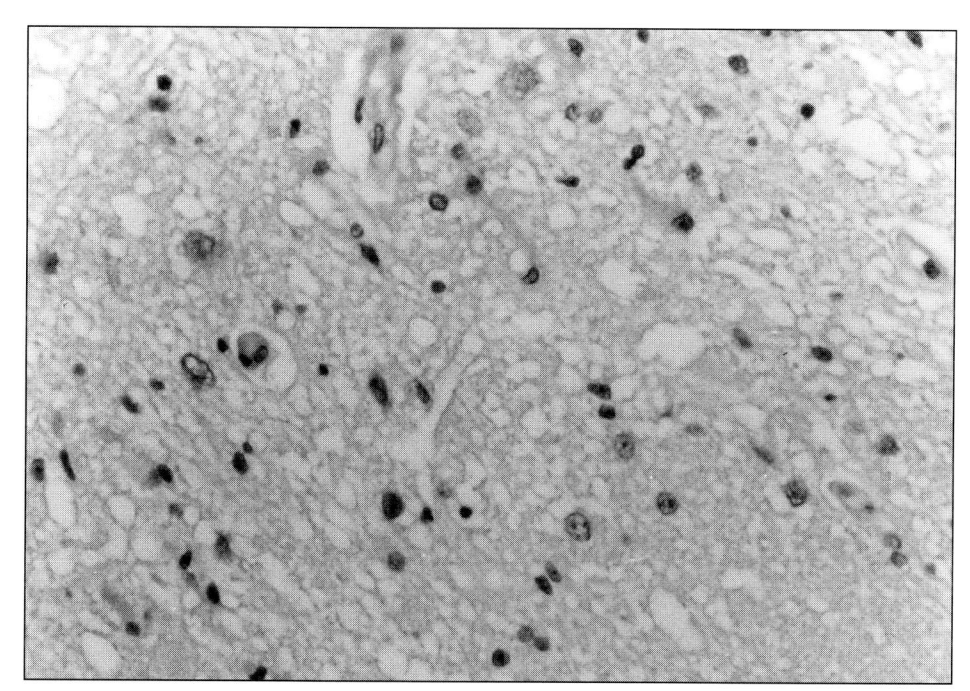

Figure 17–1. The posterior columns have subtle vacuoles in the white matter.

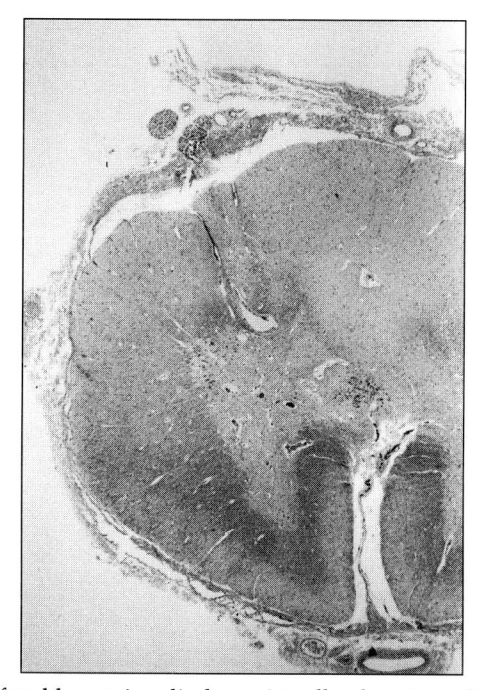

Figure 17–2. Luxol-fast blue stains disclose virtually absent myelin in the posterior and lateral columns.

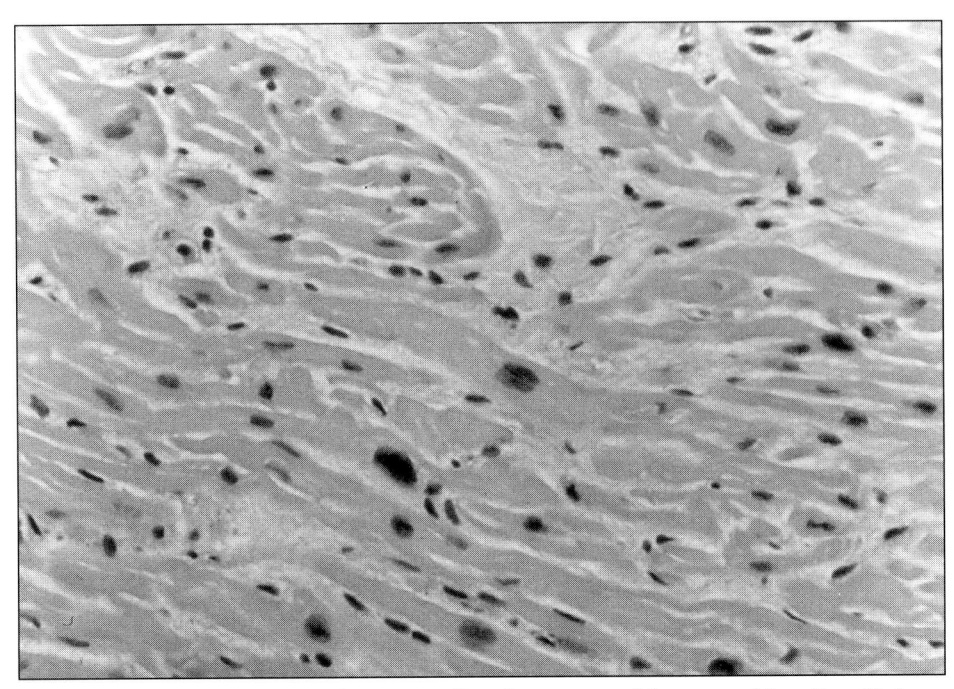

Figure 17–3. The left ventricular myocardium has scattered hypertrophic cells with large dark nuclei.

whole length of the spinal cord is involved but most severely in the cervical region. A preferential loss of the lateral part of the lateral corticospinal tract is found in the cervical spinal cord. Caudally, degeneration involves the entire lateral corticospinal tract without a medial-to-lateral gradient of involvement.[6] These tracts show loss of fibers, myelin pallor, and gliosis. Gracilis tracts are involved earlier and more severely than the cuneatus tracts. The pyramidal tracts and dorsal spinocerebellar tracts are more severely affected than the ventral cerebellar tracts. The thoracic nucleus of Clarke has neuronal loss. Anterior horn neurons may be lost, but this is not a consistent lesion. Demyelination in the pyramidal tracts and descending trigeminal roots is noted. Neuronal loss has been found in the cochlear, vestibular, glossopharyngeal, vagus, and hypoglossal nuclei. In the peripheral nervous system, lesions consist of degeneration of the posterior roots, posterior ganglia, and the peripheral nerves. Large myelinated fibers are preferentially affected.[7] Imaging studies of the spinal cord in patients with FA show decreased anteroposterior diameters of the spinal cord at C3 level. Imaging studies give abnormal signals in the posterior and lateral columns on sagittal and axial projections in most patients with FA but in none with other forms of ataxia.[8] In advanced FA, the vermis and medulla are atrophic.[9]

Patients with FA have autopsy evidence of heart disease in 100% of cases; 90% have electrocardiographic abnormalities, and 30% have clinical symptoms such as heart failure. Pathologically, the left ventricle is hypertrophic in mild cases, while the right ventricle is hypertrophic in more severe cases. Hypertrophy may be associated with dilatation. Patchy or diffuse interstitial fibrosis is usually present and fatty infiltration may be prominent.[10] Myocarditis is also common and pericardial adhesions may develop.[11] Endocardial sclerosis and mural thrombi are infrequently found. A large proportion of patients with FA have asymmetric septal hypertrophy or hypertrophic cardiomyopathy, but disarray of fibers does not occur.[12] Intramural coronary arteries may have intimal sclerosis, but the major epicardial coronary arteries are usually normal. The severity of the ataxia is not related to the severity of the cardiac findings.[10]

In one large series of all hereditary ataxias, FA accounted for almost one-third of the cases.[13] While FA is the most common and best studied of the hereditary ataxias, the differential diagnosis clinically includes the following conditions. The cerebellar heredoataxia of Marie has older age of onset, preservation of deep tendon reflexes in lower extremities, presence of spasticity, and absence of kyphoscoliosis. Familial spastic paraplegia has mild cerebellar signs associated with pyramidal signs. Abetalipoproteinemia with ataxia may actually be due to vitamin E deficiency.[1] In regard to the latter diagnosis, children with inability to absorb fat vitamins may have a similar neuropathy. Chronic cholestasis, cystic fibrosis, and abetalipoproteinemia are in this category. Significant vitamin E deficiency in these children manifests as poor myelinization.[14]

The hereditary pattern of FA is autosomal recessive but with a male preponderance. Patients with FA have a high incidence of diabetes mellitus[15] and cardiac disease with arrhythmias and congestive heart failure.[11] Considerable heterogeneity is found within families, with age of onset in some members as early as 4 years and as late as 24 years.[16] Although the gene has not yet been identified, the locus for FA was first described by Chamberlain et al in 1988 and is on chromosome 9 (9p22-cen).[17] The locus has been narrowed to a 300-kb region, but caution is urged because linkage studies are dependent on careful selection of families and limiting predictions to those with cardiomyopathy after exclusion of vitamin E deficiency.[18] The gene frequency in Spain is 1 in 127 with an incidence of 6.18 per 100,000 live births.[19] Some FA cases may have a mutation on chromosome 8.[1] Willers et al performed growth studies on fibroblasts from patients with FA. Their fibroblasts had lower plating efficiency, growth rate, and population doublings compared with normal fibroblasts.[20] These fibroblasts also had slower outgrowth of vimentin filaments and incorporated less 5-bromo-2'-deoxyuridine (BrdU) into their DNA than did normal fibroblasts.[21] Heterozygous individuals for the Friedreich's gene had fibroblasts with normal growth curves.[20]

DIAGNOSIS: Friedreich's ataxia

References

1. Ben Hamida M. Spinocerebellar heredodegeneration. In: Duckett S, ed. *Pediatric Neuropathology.* Baltimore: Williams & Wilkins; 1995:239.
2. De Michele G, Filla A, Cavalcanti F, et al. Late onset Friedreich's disease: Clinical features and mapping of mutation to the FRDA locus. *J Neurol Neurosurg Psychiatry* 1994;57:977–979.

3. Becker LE. The nervous system. In: Stocker JT, Dehner LP, ed. *Pediatric Pathology*. Philadelphia: JB Lippincott Co; 1992:459.
4. Palau F, DeMichele G, Vilchez JJ, et al. Early-onset ataxia with cardiomyopathy and retained tendon reflexes maps to the Friedreich's ataxia locus on chromosome 9q. *Ann Neurol* 1995;37:359–362.
5. Jitpimolmard S, Small J, King RH, et al. The sensory neuropathy of Friedreich's ataxia: An autopsy study of a case with prolonged survival. *Acta Neuropathol* 1993;86:29–35.
6. Murayama S, Bouldin TW, Suzuki K. Pathological study of corticospinal-tract degeneration in Friedreich's ataxia. *Neuropathol Appl Neurobiol* 1992;18:81–86.
7. Costa C, Hauw J-J. Pathology of the cerebellum, brain stem and spinal cord. In: Duckett S, ed. *Pediatric Neuropathology*. Baltimore: Williams & Wilkins; 1995:217.
8. Mascalchi M, Salvi F, Piacentini S, Bartolozzi C. Friedreich's ataxia: MR findings involving the cervical portion of the spinal cord. *AJR* 1994;163:187–191.
9. Ormerod IE, Harding AE, Miller DH, et al. Magnetic resonance imaging in degenerative ataxic disorders. *J Neurol Neurosurg Psychiatry* 1994;57:51–57.
10. Ferrans V. Metabolic and familial diseases. In: Silver MD, ed. *Cardiovascular Pathology*. 2nd ed. New York: Churchill Livingstone; 1991:1126.
11. De Girolami U, Frosch MP, Anthony DC. The central nervous system. In: Cotran RS, Kumar V, Robbins SL, ed. *Robbins Pathologic Basis of Disease*. 5th ed. Philadelphia: WB Saunders Co; 1994:1335.
12. Patterson K, Donnelly WH, Dehner LP. The cardiovascular system. In: Stocker JT, Dehner LP, ed. *Pediatric Pathology*. Philadelphia: JB Lippincott Co; 1992:609.
13. Filla A, DeMichele G, Barbieri F, Campanella G. Early onset hereditary ataxias of unknown etiology: Review of a personal series. *Acta Neurol* 1992;14:420–430.
14. Bove KE. Neuromuscular diseases. In: Stocker JT, Dehner LP, ed. *Pediatric Pathology*. Philadelphia: JB Lippincott Co; 1992:1193–1195.
15. Maertens P, Dyken PR. Neurologic degenerative diseases. In: Duckett S, ed. *Pediatric Neuropathology*. Baltimore: Williams & Wilkins; 1995:545.
16. Muller-Felber W, Rossmanith T, Spes C, Chamberlain S, Pongratz D, Deufel T. The clinical spectrum of Friedreich's ataxia in German families showing linkage to the FRDA locus on chromosome 9. *Clin Invest* 1993;71:109–114.
17. Chamberlain S, Shaw J, Rowland A, et al. Mapping of mutation causing Friedreich's ataxia to human chromosome 9. *Nature* 1988;334:248–250.
18. Monrós E, Smeyers P, Ramos MA, Prieto F, Palau F. Prenatal diagnosis of Friedreich ataxia: Improved accuracy by using new genetic flanking markers. *Prenat Diagn* 1995;15:551–554.
19. Lopez-Arlandis JM, Vilchez JJ, Palau F, Seville T. Friedreich's ataxia: An epidemiological study in Valencia. *Neuroepidemiology* 1995;14:14–19.
20. Willers I, Koeppen A, Singh S, Goedde HW. Growth studies on fibroblasts of patients with autosomal recessive Friedreich's ataxia. *Pathobiology* 1991;59:357–360.
21. Willers I, Ressler B, Singh S, Koeppen AH. Immunocytochemical studies on the vimentin distribution and cell proliferation of fibroblasts in patients with Friedreich's ataxia. *J Neurol Sci* 1993;117:159–163.

Case Eighteen

Contributed by Don B. Singer, MD
Providence, Rhode Island

History

This 11-year-old boy was admitted with severe frontal headache and confusion. His history included tonsillectomy and adenoidectomy at age 5 years with repeated removal at age 6 years. He weighed 160 pounds. His temperature was 102°F, he had dry lips, photophobia, and a heart rate of 196/minute. A sample of his cerebrospinal fluid had five mononuclear cells and one neutrophil, glucose 3.1 mmol/L, protein 240 mg/L. The serum ammonia level was 52.8 µmol/L. His course was one of rapid deterioration with progressive bradycardia and death 24 hours after admission.

Dr Singer: The thyroid gland weighs 46 g (normal 15 g at age 12 years, 20 to 25 g in adults[1]) and is obviously grossly enlarged. It has a smooth capsular surface and pink-red cut surface. Follicles are lined by hyperplastic cells with infolding into the lumens forming so-called pseudopapillae. Many follicles are apparently filled with the hyperplastic cells (Figure 18–1). Colloid is scanty and vacuolated at the periphery (Figure 18–2). Cytologically the follicle cells are tall with hyperchromatic nuclei in a basal or midcellular position. Cytoplasm is frequently vacuolated. Groups of follicle cells have eosinophilic cytoplasm and central to slightly eccentric hyperchromatic nuclei. These follicles contain no colloid. Scattered through the thyroid gland are lymphoid infiltrates (Figure 18–3).

The heart was enlarged (336 g vs 250 g expected normal weight) and had focally hypertrophic fibers with rectangular hyperchromatic nuclei. The thymus was greatly enlarged (76 g vs 15 g expected normal weight) and had hyperplastic lymphoid elements. The lymphoid tissues throughout the body were prominent with large active germinal centers. Fatty change was noted in the myocardial fibers, hepatocytes, and renal tubular epithelial cells.

Headache, confusion, and coma in a preadolescent boy were the clinical problems. These symptoms together with tachycardia, fever, and rapid progression to cardiovascular collapse raised the suspicion of Reye syndrome, but the ammonia concentration was not significantly elevated, the liver was not palpably enlarged, and there was no history of aspirin ingestion. Infection of the meninges or brain was also considered a likely cause. Although the brain was swollen, no inflammation was present. Bilateral lobar pneumonia contributed to the child's demise. We concluded that undiagnosed thyrotoxicosis with thyroid storm, precipitated by pneumonia, was the cause of this child's death.

The differential diagnosis of thyrotoxicosis includes diffuse toxic hyperplasia (Graves' disease), toxic multinodular goiter (Plummer's disease), and toxic

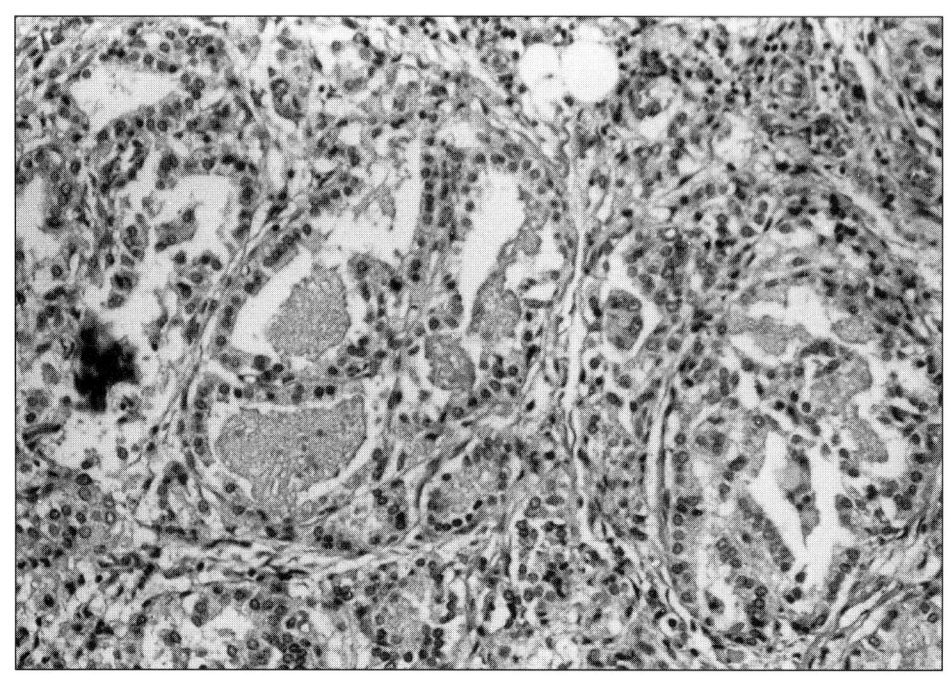

Figure 18–1. Thyroid hyperplasia with infolding of epithelium into lumens of follicles.

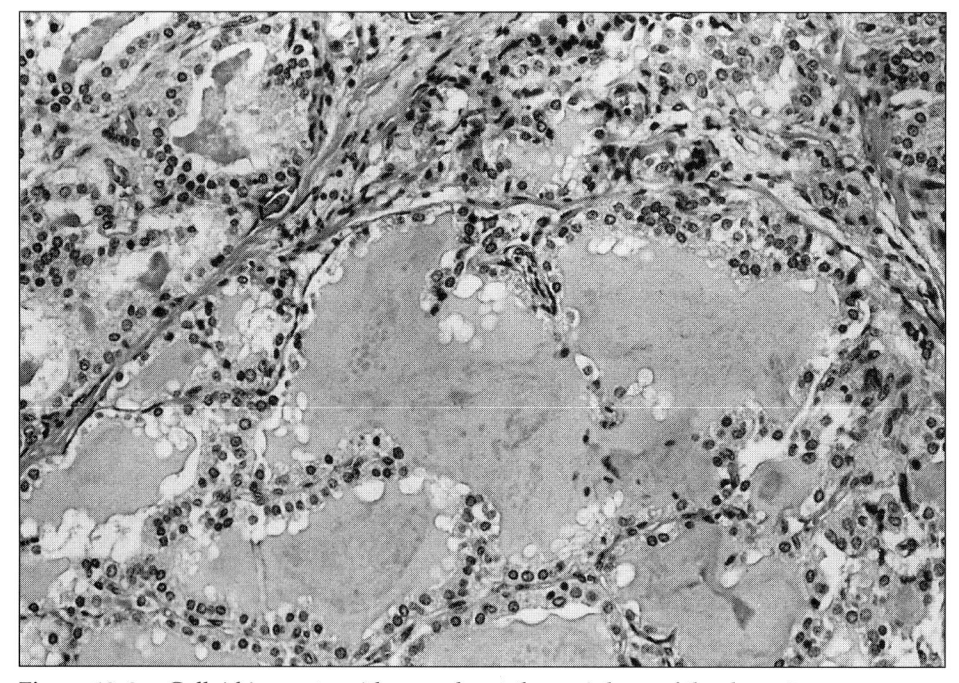

Figure 18–2. Colloid is scanty with vacuoles at the periphery of the deposits.

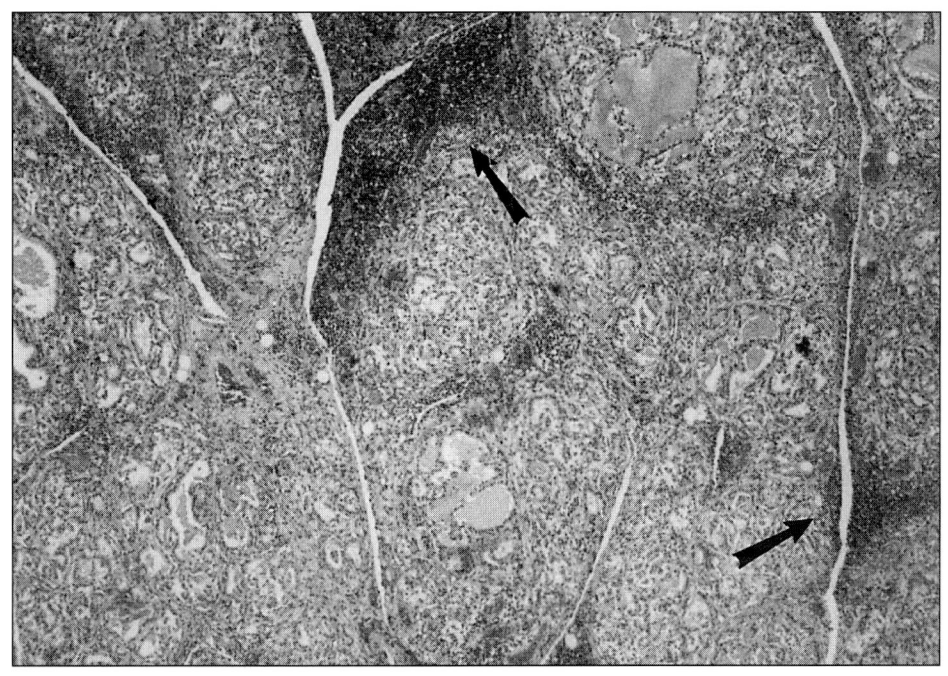

Figure 18–3. Lymphoid infiltrates (arrows) are scattered throughout the hyperplastic thyroid gland.

adenoma.[2] Rare causes include thyroiditis, hyperfunctioning thyroid carcinoma, thyroid-stimulating hormone (TSH)–secreting pituitary adenoma, choriocarcinoma or hydatidiform mole, struma ovarii, iodine-induced hyperthyroidism, and ingestion or injection of exogenous thyroid hormone.[3] All of these conditions are exceedingly rare or nonexistent in children.

In this child, the history of repeated tonsillectomy and adenoidectomy was followed by multiple myringotomies for otitis media, indicating continued obstruction of the eustachian tube by hyperplastic lymphoid tissue. Results of autopsy confirmed the presence of enlarged lymph nodes, Peyer's patches, and thymus. T-helper cells (CD4+) predominated in the dense lymphoid clusters. These cells apparently are the source of antithyroid antibodies that occur in Graves disease, i.e. the antibody that binds to the receptor for TSH and stimulates cyclic adenosine monophosphate, which results in the excessive production of thyroid hormone.[4] Cardiac hypertrophy and intracellular fat in the myocardium, hepatocytes, and renal tubules are all seen in thyrotoxicosis.[3] Other liver changes include moderate-to-mild cholestasis, lobular inflammatory infiltrate with some eosinophils, and Kupffer cell hyperplasia.[5]

In a series of 33 thyrotoxic patients who died, 13 following thyroid storm, Scheithauer et al found that pituitary glands had reduced numbers of TSH-producing cells, suggesting that elevated thyroid hormones suppressed TSH production.[6] In this child's pituitary gland, virtually no TSH-positive cells were found with immunohistochemical stains for this hormone.

About 5% of all patients with hyperthyroidism are less than 15 years of age. In children, the peak incidence occurs during adolescence, but it has been reported in fetuses, newborn infants, and children up to 2 years of age when the mothers have thyrotoxicosis.[7,8] The incidence in girls is five times that in boys. The clinical course in children is variable but usually not as fulminant as in adults. Thyroid-stimulating hormone levels are low unless there is pituitary unresponsiveness to thyroid hormones or in the more rare instance of a hypothalamic or pituitary tumor. Restlessness and nervous tremor and a voracious appetite are common. This may account for the excessive weight of this child, despite the hypermetabolic state produced by thyrotoxicosis. In pediatric patients, exophthalmos is rarely severe but may be noticeable, especially in a patient with lymphoid hyperplasia. Tachycardia, palpitations, dyspnea, cardiac enlargement, and insufficiency may endanger life.

Thyroid storm is an exaggeration of hyperthyroidism and may lead to cardiovascular collapse and death.[9] It is rare in adults and even more rare in children.[10,11] Thyroid storm has an acute onset with hyperthermia, severe tachycardia, and restlessness, often with severe headache. These features were present in the case at hand. Rapid progression to delirium, coma, and death occurs unless decisive and immediate therapy is begun.[12–14] Status epilepticus may be the presenting sign.[15] In decades past, the fatality rate from thyroid storm was 100%[16] and today, even with vigorous treatment, fatalities occur in up to 50% of cases.[12,17] Thyroid storm requires aggressive treatment with drugs that inhibit production, release, and conversion of T4 to T3.[14,16,18]

Thyroid storm is associated with certain drugs,[19–21] including over-the-counter remedies,[22] stress, fevers, and infection.[4] Children with McCune-Albright syndrome have an increased risk of thyroid storm.[23] The exact mechanism by which individuals decompensate into thyroid storm is unknown. They may have an enhanced cellular sensitivity to either catecholamines or thyroid hormone. Catecholamines are usually in low concentrations in the sera of patients with Graves' disease.[22] Complications of thyroid storm include rhabdomyolysis with elevated serum concentrations of muscle enzymes[24] and cerebral infarcts.[25]

DIAGNOSIS: Thyroid hyperplasia in boy with undiagnosed thyrotoxicosis and thyroid storm

References

1. Ueda D. Normal volume of the thyroid gland in children. *J Clin Ultrasound* 1990;18:455–462.
2. Minegishi Y, Kumada S, Suzuki H, Kusaka H, Shimozawa K, Okaniwa M. Repetitive monomorphic ventricular tachycardia in a 4-year-old boy with toxic multinodular goiter. *Acta Paediatr Scand* 1991;80:726–731.
3. Cotran RS, Kumar V, Robbins SL. The thyroid gland. In: Cotran RS, Kumar V, Robbins SL, eds. *Robbins Pathologic Basis of Disease*. 5th ed. Philadelphia: WB Saunders Co; 1994:1121.

4. DiGeorge AM, LaFranchi S. Hyperthyroidism. In: Behrman RE, Kliegman RM, Arvin AM, eds. *Nelson Textbook of Pediatrics.* 15th ed. Philadelphia, Pa: WB Saunders Co; 1996:1600–1601.
5. Sola J, Pardo-Mindan FJ, Zozaya J, Quiroga J, Sangro B, Prieto J. Liver changes in patients with hyperthyroidism. *Liver* 1991;11:193–197.
6. Scheithauer BW, Kovacs KT, Young WF Jr, Randall RV. The pituitary gland in hyperthyroidism. *Mayo Clin Proc* 1992;67:22–26.
7. Mostoufi-Zadeh M, Weiss LM, Driscoll SG. Nonimmune hydrops fetalis: A challenge in perinatal pathology. *Hum Pathol* 1985;16:785–789.
8. Page DV, Brady K, Mitchell J, Pehrson J, Wade G. The pathology of intrauterine thyrotoxicosis: Two case reports. *Obstet Gynecol* 1988;72:479–481.
9. Roth RN, McAuliffe MJ. Hyperthyroidism and thyroid storm. *Emerg Med Clin North Am* 1989;7:873–883.
10. Gavin LA. Thyroid crises. *Med Clin North Am* 1991;75:179–193.
11. Aiello DP, DuPlessis AJ, Pattishall EG III, Kulin HE. Thyroid storm: Presenting with coma and seizures in a 3-year-old girl. *Clin Pediatr* 1989;28:571–574.
12. Laman DM, Berghout A, Endtz LJ, van der Vijver JC, Wattendorff AR. Thyroid crisis presenting as coma. *Clin Neurol Neurosurg* 1984;86:295–298.
13. Mucklow ES. Fatal thyrotoxic heart disease in a 7-year-old girl. *Pediatr Cardiol* 1990;11:229–230.
14. Brunette DD, Rothong C. Emergency department management of thyrotoxic crisis with esmolol. *Am J Emerg Med* 1991;9:232–234.
15. Safe AF, Griffiths KD, Maxwell RT. Thyrotoxic crisis presenting as status epilepticus. *Postgrad Med J* 1990;66:150–152.
16. Burch HB, Wartofsky L. Life-threatening thyrotoxicosis: Thyroid storm. *Endocrinol Metab Clin North Am* 1993;22:263–277.
17. Tietgens ST, Leinung MC. Thyroid storm. *Med Clin North Am* 1995;79: 169–184.
18. Spittle L. Diagnoses in opposition: Thyroid storm and myxedema coma. *AACN Clin Issues Crit Care Nurs* 1992;3:300–308.
19. Kidess AI, Caplan RH, Reynertson RH, Wickus G. Recurrence of 131-I induced thyroid storm after discontinuing glucocorticoid therapy. *Wis Med J* 1991;90:463–465.
20. Mulligan DC, McHenry CR, Kinney W, Esselstyn CB Jr. Amiodarone-induced thyrotoxicosis: Clinical presentation and expanded indications for thyroidectomy. *Surgery* 1993;114:1114–1119.
21. Roti E, Minelli R, Gardini E, Bianconi L, Braverman LE. Thyrotoxicosis followed by hypothyroidism in patients treated with amiodarone: A possible consequence of a destructive process in the thyroid. *Arch Intern Med* 1993;153:886–892.
22. Wilson BE, Hobbs WN. Case report: Pseudoephedrine-associated thyroid storm: Thyroid hormone-catecholamine interactions. *Am J Med Sci* 1993; 306:317–319.
23. Lawless ST, Reeves G, Bowen JR. The development of thyroid storm in a child with McCune-Albright syndrome after orthopedic surgery. *Am J Dis Child* 1992;146:1099–1102.
24. Bennett WR, Huston DP. Rhabdomyolysis in thyroid storm. *Am J Med* 1984;77:733–735.

25. Page SR, Scott AR. Thyroid storm in a young woman resulting in bilateral basal ganglia infarction. *Postgrad Med J* 1993;69:813–815.
26. Herman GE, Kanluen S, Monforte J, Husain M, Spitz WU. Fatal thyrotoxic crisis. *Am J Forensic Med Pathol* 1986;7:174–176.

Case Nineteen

Contributed by James M. Angevine, MD
Madison, Wisconsin

History

The patient was a neonate who was born by cesarean section after 33-weeks' gestation because of massive enlargement of the face that was thought to be a teratoma on ultrasound examination. The face and head were markedly distorted by a solid fleshy tumor that filled the nasal cavity, extended through the cribriform plate to form a plaque-like lesion in the anterior fossa, and infiltrated the face and neck (Figure 19–1). The baby lived for only a short period after birth.

Dr Dehner: This unfortunate infant lived but a few minutes after birth, which in a sense is merciful, given the extensive involvement by this primitive round cell neoplasm whose apparent epicenter is the head and neck region. However, virtually every organ at autopsy was grossly or microscopically involved by this predominantly malignant round cell infiltrate. There was even tumor present in the fetal vessels of the placenta (Figure 19–2). Another attribute of this neoplasm is the widespread necrosis that accompanied both the gross and microscopic foci of tumor. The tumor deposits are composed of discohesive and focally cohesive collections of primitive-appearing round cells and spindle cells (Figure 19–3). A central to slightly eccentric hyperchromatic nucleus and a rim of eosinophilic cytoplasm characterize most of the polygonal cells. However, scattered tumor cells representing 5% to 10% of the total population are notable for the presence of an apparent cytoplasmic inclusion, which accounts for the rhabdoid appearance (a large polygonal cell with an eccentric, vesicular nucleus and a filamentous or eosinophilic cytoplasmic inclusion) (Figure 19–4). Mitotic figures are focally numerous. Another feature of this neoplasm was the extensive vascular space involvement.

The differential diagnosis of this primitive congenital neoplasm includes the following possibilities from the clinical and pathologic perspectives: classic neuroblastoma, primitive neuroectodermal tumor (PNET), hematolymphoid neoplasm, alveolar rhabdomyosarcoma, and malignant rhabdoid tumor. Rhabdoid or pseudorhabdoid cells have been described in a number of other neoplasms including malignant melanoma, poorly differentiated carcinoma, rhabdomyosarcoma, desmoplastic small round cell tumor, peripheral and central PNETs, and rarely, undifferentiated neuroblastoma.[1] Immunohistochemical studies display the polyantigenic or polyphenotypic character of this neoplasm with expression for vimentin, cytokeratin, muscle-specific actin, neuron-specific enolase, and epithelial membrane antigen (Figure 19–5). The tumor cells are nonreactive for the MIC2 gene product, utilizing the HBA71 antibody. Leukocyte common antigen

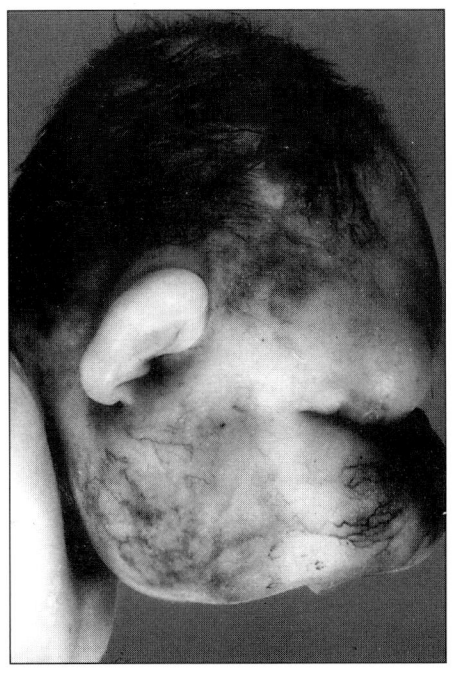

Figure 19-1. A profile view of this infant at autopsy shows a massive tumor that has infiltrated throughout the soft tissues of the facial region and into the paranasal sinuses and the base of the skull.

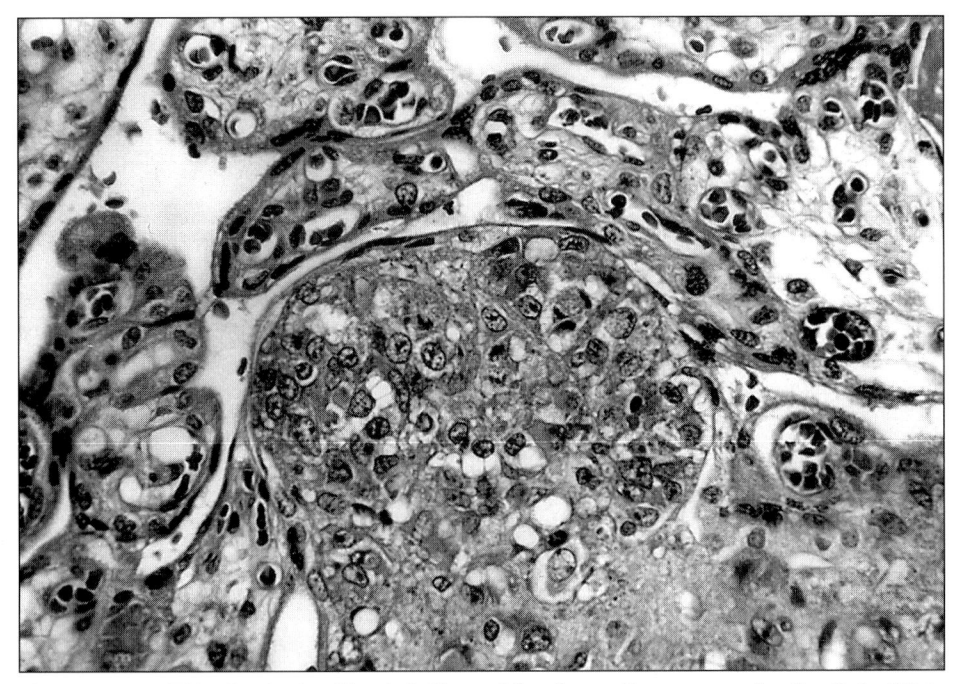

Figure 19-2. This chorionic villus is infiltrated by the malignant round cells. Only 1% to 2% of the chorionic villi contained malignant cells.

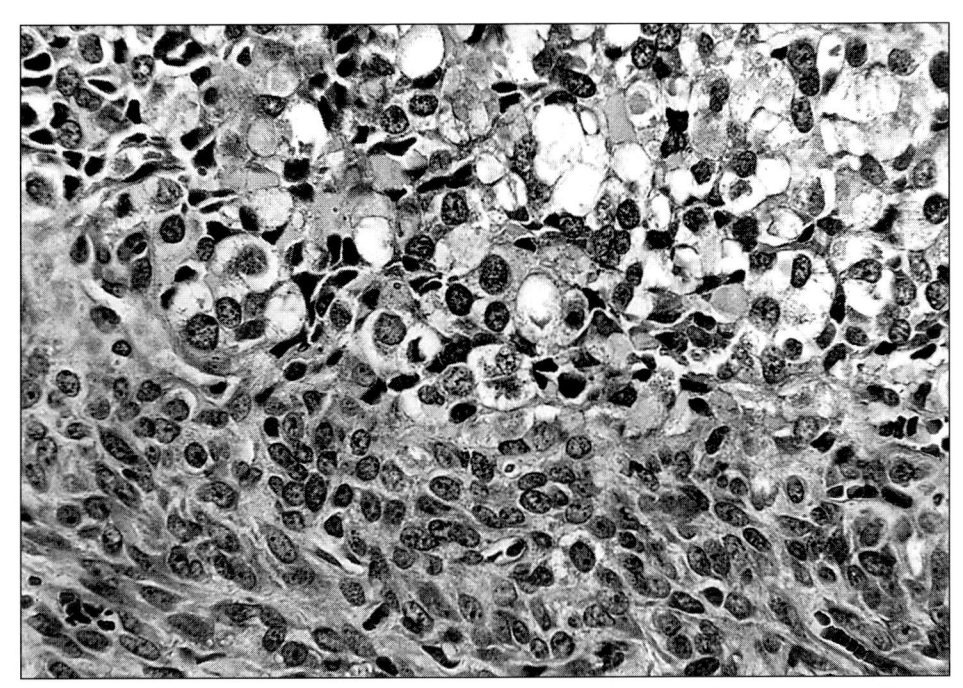

Figure 19–3. Some areas of the tumor had contiguous foci of malignant round cells and spindle cells. The nuclei of the spindle cells tended to be smaller and did not have the cytologic characteristics of rhabdoid cells.

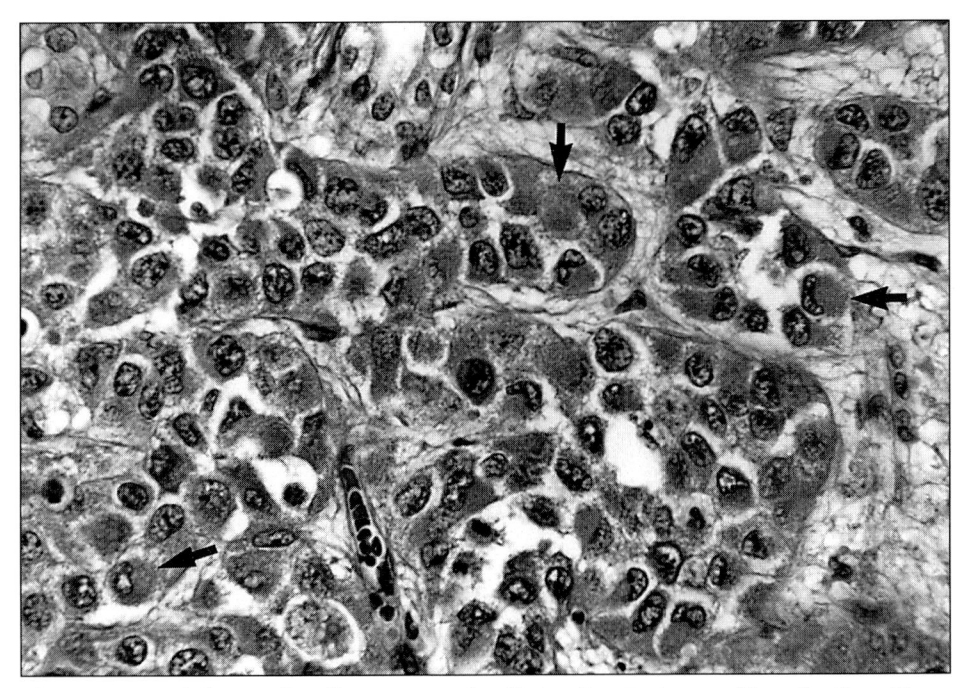

Figure 19–4. A focus of malignant round cells in discohesive profiles of cells with an alveolar appearance. The cells have a large eccentric nucleus with a prominent nucleolus, and filamentous cytoplasmic inclusions are readily apparent in some cells (arrows).

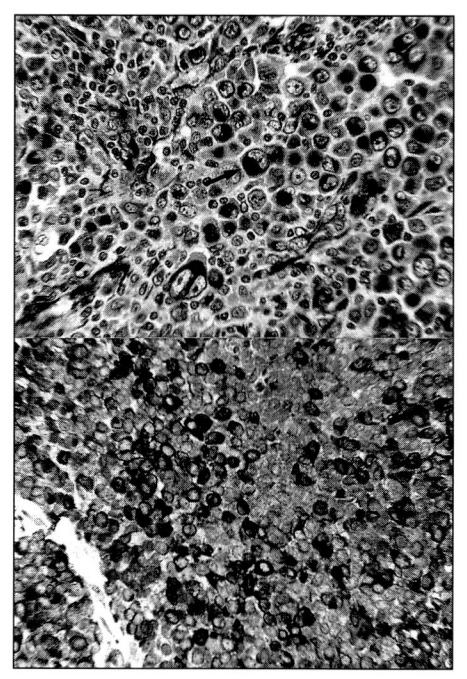

Figure 19–5. A consistent feature of rhabdoid cells in their various pathologic contexts with some exceptions in the immunohistochemical coexpression of vimentin (top) and cytoplasm (bottom). Often, one or the other of these stains highlights the filamentous inclusions as an intensely staining structure (top, arrow).

(CD45) is also nonreactive. This tumor does not have the clinical and pathologic features of classic neuroblastoma, which is the most common congenital malignant neoplasm (Table 19–1).[2–6] Both rhabdomyosarcoma and Ewing's sarcoma-PNET are excluded on the basis of the polyantigenic character and the absence of MIC2 gene product reactivity.[7] This neoplasm is regarded as a congenital malignant rhabdoid tumor that appears to have arisen in the head and neck region. The kidneys were involved by microscopic metastatic deposits in contrast to the usual presentation of a malignant renal rhabdoid tumor.[8]

It was thought at first that this neonate had a teratoma of the head and neck, which is a well-recognized category of tumors presenting in the neonatal period.[9,10] Most congenital teratomas arise in the sacrococcygeal region, but a minority of cases may present in the head and neck either as an epignathus (basisphenoid teratoma) or in the neck as a cervicothyroidal teratoma.[10] Classic neuroblastoma as a congenital neoplasm presents as either an abdominal mass or an abdominal mass with evidence of metastasis to one or more of the following sites: liver, skin and subcutis, bone marrow, and bone.[10] Congenital neuroblastoma is known to metastasize to the placenta.[11]

Since malignant rhabdoid tumor (MRT) was first described as a primary renal neoplasm of childhood, this tumor or its mimics have become recognized in a number of extrarenal sites, as a cytologic alteration in a variable number of

Table 19–1. Congenital and Connatal Neoplasms*

Tumor Type	Frequency (%)
Classic neuroblastoma	33
"Sarcoma"	33
Others	11
Renal neoplasms	6
Retinoblastoma	5
Leukemia/lymphoma	5
Brain tumor	3
Germ cell tumor	2
"Carcinoma"	1
Liver tumor	1
Total	100

*Modified from Coffin and Dehner.[10]

tumor cells in malignant mesenchymal and epithelial neoplasms and metastatic melanoma.[8,12–17] The MRT of the kidney was originally described by Beckwith and Palmer[18] as the rhabdomyosarcomatoid pattern of sarcomatous Wilms' tumor. These authors defined the histologic features of the rhabdoid tumor as "sheets of polygonal cells with abundant acidophilic cytoplasm and rounded vesicular nuclei possessing a very prominent centrally located hematoxyphilic nucleus . . . variable numbers of cells contain large, spherical, rounded hyalin, cytoplasmic masses."[8] The number of rhabdoid cells in a particular neoplasm to qualify as a MRT has been addressed by Weeks et al[8] in the following manner: "a proportion of cells with inclusions (that) varied from case to case and within individual tumors."

Histogenetic concepts and nosologic issues relating to the MRT have been discussed at length by Wick et al.[1] Basically three clinicopathologic categories of MRT are recognized: (1) malignant renal rhabdoid tumor, (2) extrarenal rhabdoid tumor, and (3) composite rhabdoid tumor. Malignant renal rhabdoid tumors comprise approximately 1.6% of all primary renal neoplasms in children; 50% of these cases present at or before 1 year of age; 13.5% of affected children have or will have a primitive neuroectodermal tumor of the brain, and the prognosis is poor with a survival of only 10% to 15%. The extrarenal rhabdoid tumor occurs more commonly in children, but the age range is considerably broader than that for the renal counterpart.[12,19] There are examples of congenital extrarenal rhabdoid tumors. The liver, brain, soft tissues, skin, uterus, and bladder are some of the primary extrarenal sites. Both histologically and immunohistochemically, the extrarenal rhabdoid tumor is virtually indistinguishable from the renal-based tumor. In contrast to the renal and extrarenal rhabdoid tumor, the composite rhabdoid tumor has a "parent" neoplasm, which is a carcinoma, sarcoma, or melanoma. These tumors occur almost exclusively in adults, and the immunophenotype tends to reflect the parent neoplasm.[20] A recent observation has been the identification of two translocations, t(11;22) and t(8;22), in MRTs, which poses the question whether MRT or at least some MRTs are representatives of the Ewing-PNET family of neoplasms.[21]

We have had the opportunity to examine one other case similar to the current one of a massive facial neoplasm in a neonate with the histologic features of MRT. Lin et al[22] reported a case of congenital extraskeletal Ewing's sarcoma of the face in an infant female who died of tumor at 3 months of age; this case is not well documented as a Ewing's sarcoma since the vimentin was negative and HBA71 or 013 was not performed. Mitchell et al[23] reported a disseminated PNET in a neonate that may have arisen in the central nervous system.

DIAGNOSIS: Malignant rhabdoid (pseudorhabdoid) tumor

References

1. Wick MR, Ritter JH, Dehner LP. Malignant rhabdoid tumor: A clinicopathologic review and conceptual discussion. *Semin Diagn Pathol* 1995;12: 233–248.
2. Harms D. Cancer in the first year of life: Pathology report from the Kiel Pediatric Tumor Registry. *Gaslini* 1990;22:115–121.
3. Salloum E, Flamant F, Caillaud JM, et al. Diagnostic and therapeutic problems of soft tissue tumors other than rhabdomyosarcoma in infants under 1 year of age. *Med Pediatr Oncol* 1990;18:37–43.
4. Carli M, Grotto P, Perilongo G, Cordero di Montezemolo G, et al. Soft tissue sarcoma in infants less than 1 year old. *Contrib Oncol* 1990;41:165–173.
5. Campbell AN, Chan HSL, O'Brien A, et al. Malignant tumours in the neonate. *Arch Dis Child* 1987;62:19–23.
6. Werb D, Scurry J, Ostor A, et al. Survey of congenital tumours in perinatal autopsies. *Pathology* 1992;24:247–253.
7. Dehner LP. Primitive neuroectodermal tumor and Ewing's sarcoma. *Am J Surg Pathol* 1993;17:1–13.
8. Weeks DA, Beckwith JB, Mierau GW, Luckey DW. Rhabdoid tumor of kidney: A report of 111 cases from the National Wilms' Tumor Study Pathology Center. *Am J Surg Pathol* 1989;13:439–458.
9. Isaacs H Jr. *Tumors of the Newborn and Infant*. St Louis: Mosby; 1991:14–16.
10. Coffin CM, Dehner LP. Congenital tumors. In: Stocker JT, Dehner LP, eds. *Pediatric Pathology*. Philadelphia: JB Lippincott; 1992:325–354.
11. Mutz ID, Stering R. Konnatales neuroblastom und plazentametastasen. *Monat Kinderheilkd* 1991;139:154–156.
12. Parham DM, Weeks DA, Beckwith JB. The clinicopathologic spectrum of putative extrarenal rhabdoid tumors: An analysis of 42 cases studied with immunohistochemistry or electron microscopy. *Am J Surg Pathol* 1994;18: 1010–1029.
13. Gururangan S, Bowman LC, Parham DM, et al. Primary extracranial rhabdoid tumors: Clinicopathologic features and response to ifosfamide. *Cancer* 1993;71:2653–2659.
14. Hanna SL, Langston JW, Parham DM, Douglass EC. Primary malignant rhabdoid tumor of the brain: Clinical, imaging, and pathologic findings. *AJNR* 1993;14:107–115.

15. Ushigome S, Shimoda T, Nikaido T, Takasaki S. Histopathologic, diagnostic and histogenetic problems in malignant soft tissue tumor: Reassessment of malignant fibrous histiocytoma, epithelioid sarcoma, malignant rhabdoid tumor, and neuroectodermal tumor. *Acta Pathol Jpn* 1992;42:691–706.
16. Tsuenyoshi M, Daimaru Y, Hashimoto H, Enjoji M. Malignant soft tissue neoplasms with the histologic features of renal rhabdoid tumors: An ultrastructural and immunohistochemical study. *Hum Pathol* 1985;16:1235–1242.
17. Chang ES, Wick MR, Swanson PE, Dehner LP. Metastatic malignant melanoma with "rhabdoid" features. *Am J Clin Pathol* 1994;102:426–431.
18. Beckwith JB, Palmer NF. Histopathology and prognosis of Wilms' tumors: Results from the National Wilms' Tumor Study. *Cancer* 1978;41:1937–1948.
19. Okada A, Takehara H, Masamune K, et al. A newborn case of extrarenal malignant rhabdoid tumor. *Tokushima J Exper Med* 1993;40:109–112.
20. Mount SL, Lee KR, Taatjes DJ. Carcinosarcoma (malignant mixed müllerian tumor) of the uterus with a rhabdoid tumor component. An immunohistochemical, ultrastructural, and immunoelectron microscopic case study. *Am J Clin Pathol* 1995;103:235–239.
21. Newsham I, Daub D, Besnard-Guerin C, Cavenee W. Molecular sublocalization and characterization of the 11;22 translocation breakpoint in a malignant rhabdoid tumor. *Genomics* 1994;19:433–440.
22. Lim TC, Tan WTL, Lee YS. Congenital extraskeletal Ewing's sarcoma of the face: A case report. *Head Neck* 1994;16:75–78.
23. Mitchell CS, Wood BP, Shimada H. Neonatal disseminated primitive neuroectodermal tumor. *AJR* 1994;162:1160.

Case Twenty

Contributed by Louis P. Dehner, MD
St Louis, Missouri

History

The patient is a 14-year-old girl with a rapidly enlarging mass over the course of several days. A biopsy and complete excision were performed. Postoperatively, she received chemotherapy (Ewing's sarcoma protocol) and irradiation therapy. She has been tumor-free in the 8-month interval since the diagnosis.

Dr Dehner: This tumor of the vulva measured approximately 2 cm in greatest dimension and had a circumscribed, somewhat multinodular appearance. The tumor had a gray-tan to white, mucoid surface with small areas of hemorrhage. Microscopically, the tumor has a variable growth pattern consisting of diffuse areas and lobular to nodular foci, with a relatively uniform cellular appearance (Figure 20–1). Incomplete dense fibrous septa partially surround groups of tumor cells in the lobular areas. There are also foci of necrosis; cuffs of tumor cells in these areas surround vascular structures (Figure 20–2). This neoplasm qualifies cytologically as a "malignant small-cell tumor." The tumor cells are crowded, but in most areas the cells have retained a monolayer-like growth rather than haphazardly arranged, overlapping nuclei (Figure 20–3). The nuclei are round to slightly ovoid and have delicate chromatin and one or more micronucleoli. Mitotic figures are moderately abundant. Rosette-like profiles were suggested in some areas, but true rosettes were not apparent.

A neoplasm with this histologic appearance, in this anatomic site, and in an adolescent is rhabdomyosarcoma, primitive neuroectodermal tumor (PNET) or Ewing's sarcoma (EWS). The growth pattern and zonal necrosis tend to exclude a hematopoietic malignancy and a classic neuroblastoma is highly unlikely, even as a metastasis, in a patient of this age. One could possibly argue that a metastasis from a small-cell carcinoma of the cervix or ovary should be considered for reasons of completeness. The possibility of rhabdomyosarcoma, in particular the alveolar variant, is a logical first choice; some of the features displayed by this neoplasm could be explained on the basis of a rhabdomyosarcoma, but the growth pattern and cytologic features are more like an embryonal rhabdomyosarcoma than an alveolar rhabdomyosarcoma. One generally does not encounter the exquisite lobular growth noted in this case in an alveolar rhabdomyosarcoma, but it is seen with some regularity in an embryonal rhabdomyosarcoma. Large, anaplastic cells with eosinophilic cytoplasm were not seen in this neoplasm, whose presence in a malignant round cell neoplasm is highly provocative for an alveolar rhabdomyosarcoma. The vimentin and 013 immunostains are strongly positive (Figure 20–4, top and bottom). Muscle-

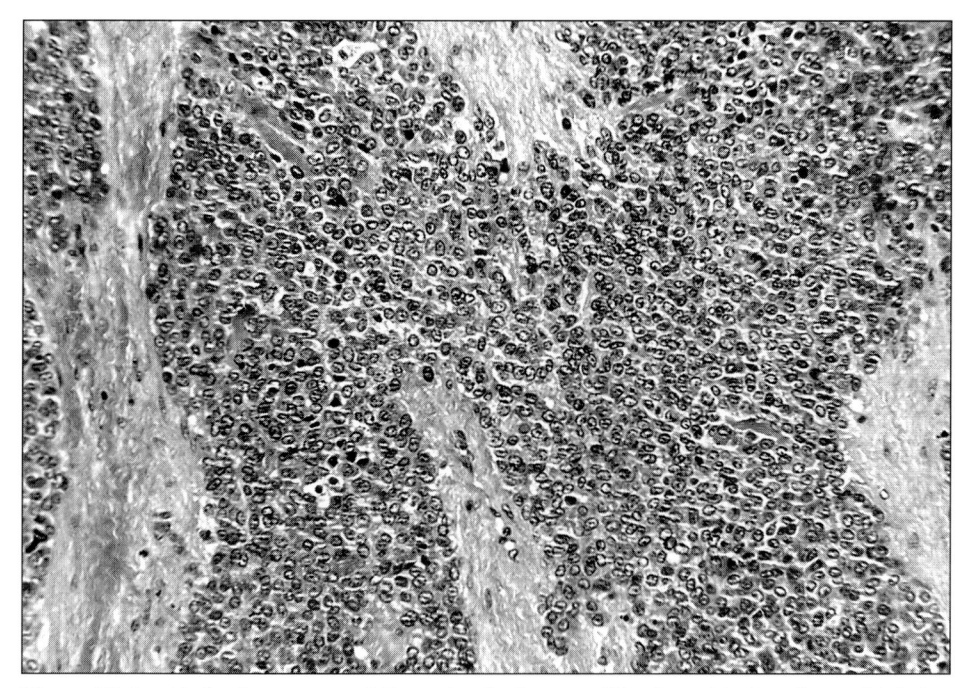

Figure 20–1. Ewing's sarcoma of the vulva is shown with a broad trabecular and lobular pattern of growth. Fibrous septa are prominent in areas of the tumor with this microscopic appearance.

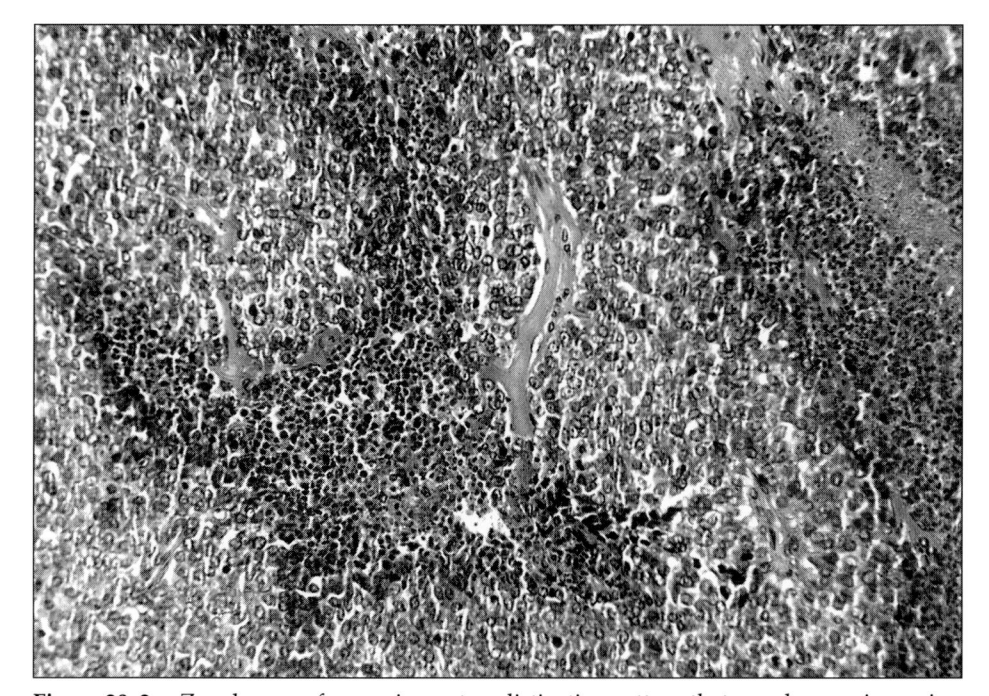

Figure 20–2. Zonal areas of necrosis create a distinctive pattern that may be seen in a primitive neuroectodermal tumor, classic neuroblastoma, retinoblastoma, and neuroendocrine carcinoma.

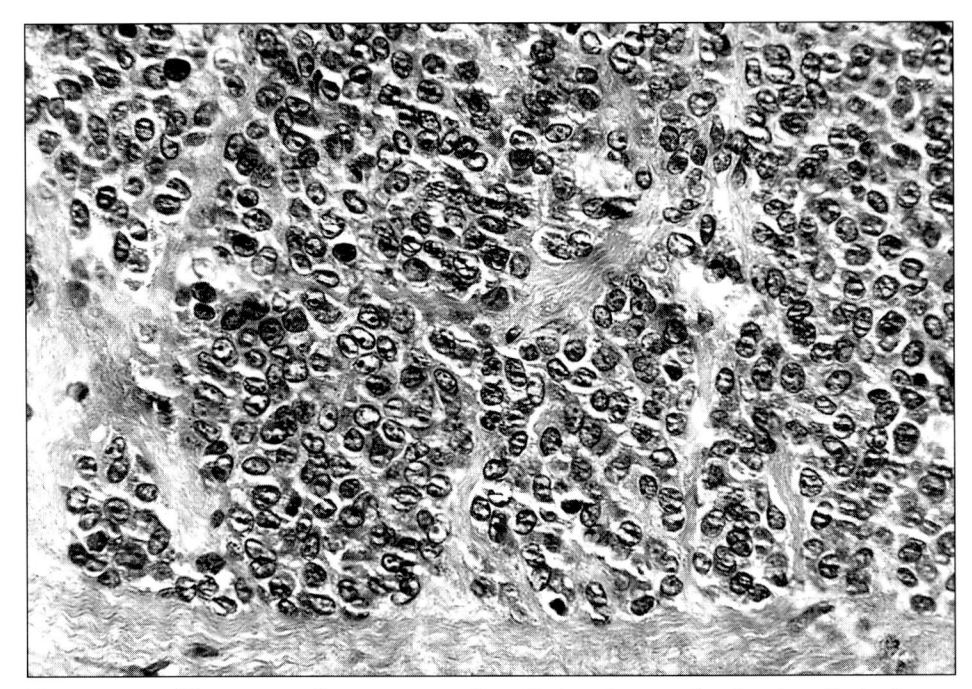

Figure 20–3. The tumor cells are more or less distinct from each other in a Ewing's sarcoma, whereas the cells in a primitive neuroectodermal tumor tend to be more crowded. Many tumor cells in this focus appear to have a clear space around the nucleus representing the glycogen-filled cytoplasm.

specific actin, desmin, and S-100 protein immunostains were nonreactive in the tumor cell population. This tumor also shows focal periodic acid–Schiff–positivity, which was diastase digestible.

Our interpretation of this neoplasm is EWS of soft tissues since it did not have rosette formation but had the delicate nuclear chromatin and the more or less monolayer growth of an EWS.[1–3] We do not rely on the expression of "neural markers" like neuron-specific enolase, Leu-7, or S-100 protein to differentiate between EWS and PNET since they are not considered to be reliable discriminators between the two tumors. The rationale to differentiate between these two related neoplasms is based on the observations from several clinicopathologic studies that have consistently found that the prognosis for PNET is worse than that for EWS with a statistically significant difference in outcome.[4–8] Whereas 65% to 70% of patients with soft tissue EWS are long-term survivors, approximately the same percentage of patients succumb to the PNET. The presence of rosettes, high-grade nuclear morphologic features, and cellular crowding are the features of the more aggressive PNET (Table 20–1).

A substantial body of literature has established that EWS and PNET share a common balanced translocation, t(11;22)(q24;q12), or a variant translocation, t(21;22)(q22;q12), in virtually 100% of cases.[9–12] If the translocation is lacking, then one can probably conclude that the neoplasm is not a PNET or EWS. The t(11;22) translocation creates a unique fusion transcript of the EWS gene on chromosome

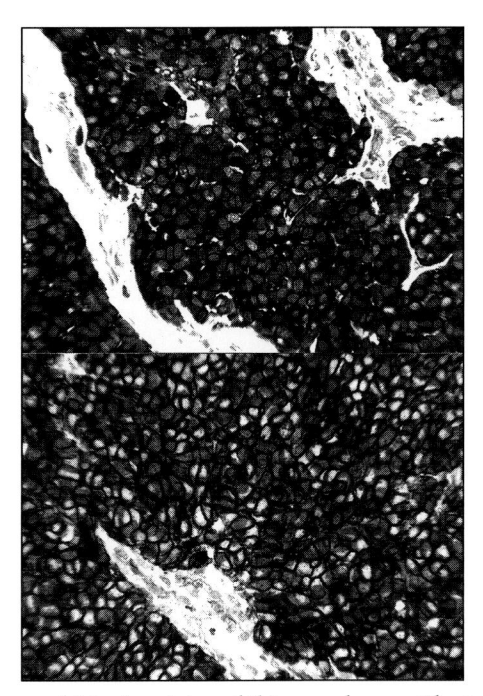

Figure 20–4. The immunohistochemistry of this neoplasm with strong cytoplasmic reactivity for vimentin (top) and intense membrane positivity for O13 (bottom) corroborate the microscopic impression of a malignant small-cell tumor in the Ewing's sarcoma–primitive neuroectodermal tumor family.

Table 20–1. Comparative Features of Primitive Neuroectodermal Tumor and Ewing's Sarcoma

	PNET	*EWS*
Pattern	Lobular and geographic	Formless sheets and/or lobular
Necrosis	Prominent and multifocal	Minimal to prominent with confluent necrosis
Rosettes	+	–
Nuclei	Overlapping, dense chromatin, round to ovoid	Monolayer, fine chromatin, uniformly round
Mitoses	Abundant, atypical	Variable, typical
Cytoplasm	Difficult to discern	Clear space around nucleus
PAS reaction	Minimal, focal or negative	Often strong
Immunohistochemistry	VIM, CK±, O13	VIM, CK±, O13

Abbreviations: PNET = primitive neuroectodermal tumor; EWS = Ewing's sarcoma; PAS = periodic acid–Schiff; VIM = vimentin; CK = cytokeratin.

22 with the Fli 1 gene, an *ets* proto-oncogene, on chromosome 11. An aberrant transcriptional activator protein that drives cellular replication is the consequence with the loss of normal feedback mechanisms to regulate cell replication.[13]

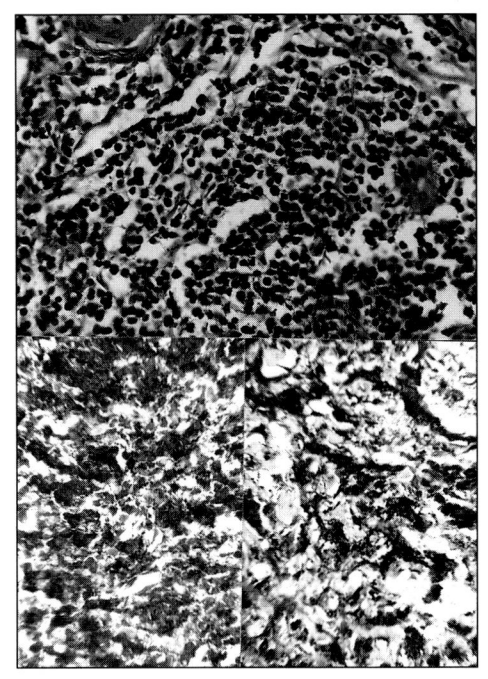

Figure 20–5. Acute lymphocytic (lymphoblastic) leukemia or lymphoblastic lymphoma may present as a solitary bone lesion mimicking Ewing's sarcoma, but these children are usually younger than those with Ewing's sarcoma. The malignant small-cell population closely resembles Ewing's sarcoma (top). These tumors are O13 immunopositive (bottom, left) like Ewing's sarcoma. Leukocyte common antigen (CD45) is expressed by this neoplasm (bottom, right), but this marker is not consistently immunoreactive in these primitive lymphoid neoplasms.

Another characteristic of EWS-PNET is the expression of the MIC2 gene product on the cell membranes, which is recognized by the antibodies HBA71, O13 or 12E7.[14–17] As far as it can be ascertained, there is no relationship between the translocation of chromosomes 11 and 22 and MIC2 expression since the latter gene is located in the pseudoautosomal region of the X and Y chromosomes. Almost 100% of PNETs and EWSs are O13 or HBA71 positive. Therefore, this marker is a highly sensitive one, but there are some specificity problems since virtually 100% of acute lymphoblastic leukemias (ALL) or lymphoblastic lymphomas are also O13 positive.[15,18] Some alveolar rhabdomyosarcomas also have membrane immunopositivity for the MIC2 gene product.[15,16] We have seen several cases of T-ALL or lymphoblastic lymphoma presenting as a solitary bone lesion that had been diagnosed originally as EWS on the basis of O13 positivity (Figure 20–5, top and bottom). As we also know, T-ALL may be a difficult neoplasm to diagnose in some cases even after a battery of immunostains.

Ewing's sarcoma and PNET are inexplicable in some of their clinical manifestations. Over 90% of EWSs present in the bone, whereas a similar proportion of PNETs are found in the soft tissues. Approximately 20% of all sarcomas in childhood are PNETs and an additional 5% of cases are EWSs.[19,20] Ewing's sarcoma of soft tissues is seen in adolescents and young adults like its osseous counterpart, but PNET may present in infancy or into late adulthood.[21] Both tumors have a predilection for the paravertebral and chest wall region. However, both of these neoplasms may present in unusual sites and circumstances, like a recent case of a renal PNET in a 17-year-old female that we have seen. Nirenberg et al[22] have reported an EWS of the vulva among 10 vulvar sarcomas. Likewise, there is a report of a PNET of the vulva.[23]

DIAGNOSIS: Soft tissue Ewing's sarcoma of the vulva

References

1. Steiner GC, Neuroectodermal tumor versus Ewing's sarcoma: Immunohistochemical and electron microscopic observations. *Curr Top Pathol* 1989;80:1–29.
2. Roessner A, Jurgens H. Round cell tumors of bone. *Pathol Res Pract* 1993;189:1111–1136.
3. Dehner LP. Primitive neuroectodermal tumor and Ewing's sarcoma. *Am J Surg Pathol* 1993;17:1–13.
4. Cavazzana AO, Ninfo V, Roberts J, Triche TJ. Peripheral neuroepithelioma: A light microscopic, immunocytochemical, and ultrastructural study. *Mod Pathol* 1992;5:71–78.
5. Miser JS, Kinsella TJ, Triche TJ, et al. Treatment of peripheral neuroepithelioma in children and young adults. *J Clin Oncol* 1987;5:1752–1758.
6. Marina NM, Etcubanas E, Parham DM, et al. Peripheral primitive neuroectodermal tumor (peripheral neuroepithelioma) in children. *Cancer* 1989;64:1952–1960.
7. Schmidt D, Herrmann C, Jurgen SH, Harms D. Malignant peripheral neuroectodermal tumor and its necessary distinction from Ewing's sarcoma. *Cancer* 1991;68:2251–2259.
8. Kushner BH, Hajdu SI, Gulati SC, et al. Extracranial primitive neuroectodermal tumor. *Cancer* 1991;67:1825–1829.
9. Turc-Carel C, Aurias A, Mugneret F, et al. Chromosomes in Ewing's sarcoma: I, An evaluation of 85 cases and remarkable consistency of t(11;22)(q24;q12). *Cancer Genet Cytogenet* 1988;32:229–238.
10. Delattre O, Zucman J, Melot T, et al. The Ewing family of tumors: a subgroup of small-round-cell tumors defined by specific chimeric transcripts. *N Engl J Med* 1994;331:294–299.
11. Sorensen PHB, Lessnick SL, Lopez-Terrada D, et al. A second Ewing's sarcoma translocation, t(21;22), fuses the EWS gene to another ETS-family transcription factor, ERG. *Nature Genet* 1994;6:146–151.
12. Ladanyi M. The emerging molecular genetics of sarcoma translocations. *Diagn Mol Pathol* 1995;4:162–173.
13. Ohno T, Ouchida M, Lee L, et al. The EWS gene, involved in Ewing family of tumors, malignant melanoma of soft parts and desmoplastic small round cell tumors, codes for an RNA binding protein with novel regulatory domains. *Oncogene* 1994;9:3087–3097.

14. Dierick AMN, Roels H, Langlois M. The immunophenotype of Ewing's sarcoma. An immunohistochemical analysis. *Pathol Res Pract* 1993;189:26–32.
15. Weidner N, Tjoe J. Immunohistochemical profile of monoclonal antibody 013: Antibody that recognizes glycoprotein p30/32 MIC2 and is useful in diagnosing Ewing's sarcoma and peripheral neuroepithelioma. *Am J Surg Pathol* 1994;18:486–494.
16. Ambros IM, Ambros PF, Strehl S, et al. MIC2 is a specific marker for Ewing's sarcoma and peripheral primitive neuroectodermal tumor. *Cancer* 1991;67:1886–1893.
17. Perlman EJ, Dickman PS, Askin FB, et al. Ewing's sarcoma: Routine diagnostic utilization of MIC2 analysis: A Pediatric Oncology Group/Children's Cancer Group Intergroup Study. *Hum Pathol* 1994;25:304–307.
18. Riopel M, Dickman PS, Link MP, Perlman EJ. MIC2 analysis in pediatric lymphomas and leukemias. *Hum Pathol* 1994;25:396–399.
19. Harms D. Soft tissue sarcomas in the Kiel Pediatric Tumor Registry. *Curr Top Pathol* 1995;89:31–45.
20. Shimada H, Newton WA Jr, Soule EH, et al. Pathologic features of extraosseous Ewing's sarcoma: A report from the Intergroup Rhabdomyosarcoma Study. *Hum Pathol* 1988;19:442–453.
21. Lee CS, Southey MC, Slater H, et al. Primary cutaneous Ewing's sarcoma/peripheral primitive neuroectodermal tumors in childhood. A molecular, cytogenetic, and immunohistochemical study. *Diagn Mol Pathol* 1995;4:174–181.
22. Nirenberg A, Ostor AG, Slavin J, et al. Primary vulvar sarcomas. *Int J Gynecol Pathol* 1995;14:55–62.
23. Scherr GR, d'Ablaing G, Ovzounian JM. Peripheral primitive neuroectodermal tumor of the vulva. *Gynecol Oncol* 1994;54:254–258.